Copyright © 2021 -All rights reserved.

No part of this book may be reproduced or transmitted in any form or by any means, electronic or mechanical, including photocopying and recording, or by any information storage and retrieval system, without permission in writing from the publisher. This is a work of fiction. Names, places, characters and incidents are either the product of the author's imagination or are used fictitiously, and any resemblance to any actual persons, living or dead, organizations, events or locales is entirely coincidental. The unauthorized reproduction or distribution of this copyrighted work is ilegal.

Please note the information contained within this document is for educational and entertainment purposes only. All effort has been executed to present accurate, up to date, reliable, complete information. No warranties of any kind are declared or implied. Readers acknowledge that the author is not engaged in the rendering of legal, financial, medical, or professional advice. The content within this book has been derived from various sources. Please consult a licensed professional before attempting any techniques outlined in this book. By reading this document, the reader agrees that under no circumstances is the author responsible for any losses, direct or indirect, that are incurred as a result of the use of the information contained within this document, including, but not limited to, errors, omissions, or inaccuracies.

CONTENTS

INTRODUCTION 4

CHAPTER 1: OVERVIEW OF CARBOHYDRATES.................................9

CHAPTER 2: BASICS OF CARB CYCLING 17

CHAPTER 3: CARB CYCLING VS OTHER DIETS............................22

CHAPTER 4: CARB CYCLING, INSULIN RESISTANCE AND DIABETES 36

CHAPTER 5: HOW TO GET STARTED ON THE CARB CYCLING DIET...................41

CHAPTER 6: BEST FOODS FOR THE CARB CYCLING DIET 44

CHAPTER 7: CARB CYCLING-FRIENDLY BREAKFAST RECIPES 50

    Low Carb..50

        Bacon & Eggs..50

        Baked Eggs With Tex-Mex Beef Casserole 52

        Frittata With Spinach 54

        Banana Waffles 56

    Moderate Carb...58

        Heavy Breakfast With Fried Eggs and Yogurt 58

        Chickpea Flour Pancakes...60

        Banana Egg Pancakes 62

    High Carb...63

        Dutch Apple Pancake...63

        Ironman Oatmeal 65

        Carrot Cake Protein Oatmeal 66

CHAPTER 8: CARB CYCLING-FRIENDLY LUNCH/DINNER RECIPES 67

    Low Carb..67

        Cheesy Chicken and Rice 67

        Santa Fe Chicken 69

        Indian Chicken Skillet 71

        Sesame Ginger Beef With Noodles 73

    Moderate Carb...75

        Harira 75

        Carrot, Ginger and Lentil Soup..78

        Pea and Ham Soup With Salami Pesto Puff Pastry 80

    High Carb...82

Lentil and Brown Rice Salad 82

Char Siu Beef With Broccolini 84

Sake Chicken With Buckwheat Noodles... 86

CHAPTER 9: CARB CYCLING-FRIENDLY SNACKS 88

Low Carb.. 88

Salt and Vinegar Zucchini Chips 88

Easy Granola.. 90

Strawberry Cream Cheese Cups 92

Parmesan Cheese Chips 93

Moderate Carb... 94

Soft Pretzels.. 94

Peanut Butter Coconut Cookies 96

Plantains With Cinnamon... 98

High Carb.. 100

The Recovery Sandwich 100

Shrimp and Lemon Pasta... 102

Banana Muffins 104

APPENDIX : RECIPES INDEX... 106

INTRODUCTION

Not having enough time in the day due to busy schedules, coupled with the convenience of buying take-out meals, has led to a high consumption of sugar, salt, and calories, with inadequate intake of fresh fruit and vegetables. If we look at a typical American diet, it shows that 75 percent of the population doesn't eat enough food containing healthy oils, vegetables, dairy and fruit. However, more than half exceed the total protein and grain food recommendations. They are eating excessive levels of refined grains instead of whole grains. As for protein, people are eating too much red meat and not much seafood. Most Americans also exceed the recommended amounts of sodium, saturated fats and added sugars (Dietary Guidelines for Americans 8th Edition, 2015). A big portion of the typical diet includes "convenience" foods, which come from restaurants or fast-food chains, are store-bought, processed, and packaged. They come with unhealthy amounts of sodium, calories, sugar and fat. Packaged and processed food are not just convenient, they are also cheaper compared to fresh fruits and vegetables and lean meats. Because of these unhealthy eating practices, we've seen an upswing of people diagnosed with chronic diseases relating to diets such as some cancers, obesity, cardiovascular diseases, diabetes and hypertension.

Unfortunately, most people only become motivated to become more aware and educated about proper nutrition after they have been diagnosed with a chronic disease. At this point, they learn how to read food labels to make better decisions. Once diagnosed with a chronic disease, people get access to health professionals such as nutritionists, dieticians, and even the doctors themselves who teach them proper nutrition to manage their disease and what food to avoid.

Data from a recent National Health and Nutrition Examination Survey showed that those who habitually read food labels consumed less sugar, saturated fat, and fewer calories and had more fiber intake in their diet than those who don't (Chen et al., 2011). And those who have a healthier diet live longer and lower their risks of these diet-related chronic diseases. Rather than wait, let's start your journey towards better health today.

Chronic Diseases From Poor Nutrition

Overweight and Obesity

Having a healthy diet, along with getting enough sleep and exercise, prevents you from gaining extra pounds. Obesity opens the doors to various chronic diseases, which is why it is important to control your weight. Poor nutrition arises from eating food with empty calories or few nutrients. When you eat food that isn't good for you, you tend to eat more than if you were eating nutritionally-dense food. As a result, you consume more calories than your body can burn. The calories are then stored as fat, and that's how you gain weight. As you can see from the list of chronic diseases below, most, if not all, are due to the strain of being overweight or obese, illustrating just how important it is to maintain a healthy weight. Diet or exercise cannot prevent obesity on their own. To keep weight at a healthy level, you need to make sure that you eat healthy food, get enough exercise and get enough sleep.

Stroke and Heart Disease

According to guidelines, it is recommended that sodium intake should not exceed 2,300 mg per day. To compare, the average American diet includes 3,400 mg of sodium in a day. Seventy percent of the sodium comes from food that is restaurant- or store-bought, processed or packaged (*Poor Nutrition*, 2019). Consuming too much sodium leads to an increase in blood pressure, which subsequently puts you at risk for stroke and heart disease.

Having a high level of cholesterol also increases this risk, due to the hardening of arteries from plaque.

Being overweight and obese also increases your chances of getting a heart attack. Compared to people of average weight, those who are overweight by 5 to 15 percent have more than twice the number of deaths from heart attacks. For those who are overweight by 25 percent or more, the number jumps to 5 times higher than average (Ikeda, 1993). If you happen to be diabetic and suffer from a heart attack or stroke, the chances of it being fatal increases up to three times as much.

Carrying extra pounds is also connected to having high blood pressure, but it's more due to the waist-to-hip ratios than to the weight itself. Those with lower waist-to-hip ratios have a lower blood pressure than those who have higher waist-to-hip ratios.

Type 2 Diabetes

Extra weight increases a person's chances of developing type 2 diabetes because, over time, their bodies become insulin resistant. It is very important for someone who is prediabetic or diabetic to watch their sugar intake to prevent spikes. Having too much glucose in their blood for long periods leads to damage to many organs in the body.

The risk of developing type 2 diabetes doubles for those who are 20 percent overweight. In fact, the risk keeps doubling for every additional 20 percent weight gain. Similar to high blood pressure, having a higher waist-to-hip ratio increases your chances of developing this disease. The best way to keep your blood sugar under control is to lose weight to improve your body's ability to process glucose.

Gallstones

The most common type of gallstone is composed of cholesterol and forms small, hard pellets that block the bile duct. This causes intense pain on the upper right and center of your abdomen, in the back pain or pain in the right shoulder. Nausea and vomiting could also occur.

Being overweight makes your liver produce more cholesterol, leading to gallstones. They are yellow in color and usually consist of undissolved cholesterol. Other causes could possibly be when your bile has too much bilirubin, which is a chemical produced when red blood cells are broken down. Blood disorders, biliary tract infections and cirrhosis can be the cause of your liver producing too much bilirubin. Gallstones formed from excessive bilirubin are called pigment gallstones and are dark brown or black. Another cause of gallstones could be when your gallbladder doesn't empty completely or frequently enough, which concentrates bile and forms gallstones. Those who experience symptoms of gallstones usually require surgery to have the organ removed.

Having gallstones can cause cholecystitis or inflammation of your gallbladder. Bile duct infection and jaundice can also occur when the gallstones block the common bile duct. If these stones block the pancreatic duct, pancreatitis, or inflammation of the pancreas occurs. Those who have a history of gallstones can develop cancer of this organ, but the chances of this occurring are very small.

You can minimize the risk of developing gallstones by keeping a healthy weight. If you are overweight or obese, lose weight slowly (about 1 to 2 pounds a week), as rapid weight loss increases your chances of developing painful gallstones. Eat foods that are high in fiber and don't skip meals.

Cancer

Being overweight or obese also increases your chances of developing at least 13 types of cancer, including colorectal cancer, breast cancer and endometrial cancer. These three cancers make up 40 percent of diagnosed cancers (*Poor Nutrition*, 2019).

Asthma

While a poor diet does not cause asthma, one study showed that a poor diet increases the severity of an asthma attack (Walker, n.d.). There is also some evidence that shows those who have diets higher in omega-3 fatty acids, vitamins C and E, selenium, beta-carotene, magnesium and flavonoids have lower occurrences of asthma. The same is true for those who grew up eating a Mediterranean-style diet, which is a diet that limits the consumption of red meat and a moderate amount of dairy, and a daily intake of healthy oils and fats, vegetables, whole grains, and whole fruits, as well as weekly consumption of eggs, fish, poultry, and beans.

Other studies show teens with poor nutrition will most likely have symptoms of asthma and those who are deficient in omega-3 fatty acids and vitamins C and E will most likely have poor lung function (Ambardekar, 2020).

Severe asthma can be linked to obesity, so it is important to keep a healthy weight if you're asthmatic.

While there is no direct link between asthma and nutrition, it doesn't hurt to make sure you eat a healthy diet anyway.

Parkinson's Disease

Some studies in mice show that obesity increases the chances of developing Parkinson's Disease due to an increase in the growth of α-synuclein clumps (Walker, n.d.). There is no diet specific to those suffering from Parkinson's Disease. They are encouraged to maintain good health and consume a balanced diet consisting of complex carbohydrates, protein and healthy fats.

Deficiency in Brain Function

The human brain develops the fastest from conception to the second birthday. It is important to maintain a healthy diet full of iron and folate while pregnant, to aid in the brain development of the baby, as well as providing a balanced diet to the child after birth.

Mental Health

Aside from affecting the body, unhealthy diets also impact the brain. Those who have diets high in refined sugars and saturated fats have more occurrences of anxiety, depressive symptoms and depression. A poor diet is connected to having a smaller left hippocampus, which is responsible for mood regulation and depression, memory and learning. In rats, those who had diets high in sugar and fat, even for short-term consumption, resulted in impaired memory and learning (Walker, n.d.).

CHAPTER 1: OVERVIEW OF CARBOHYDRATES

Carbohydrates are a macronutrient that your body needs daily – along with protein and fat.

Carbohydrates need to be part of our diet because they help our bodies function well. They are the primary source of energy for our body and organs, aiding in physical performance, recovery and muscle building. Carbohydrates also help you with mood swings and self-control. Have you noticed, for example, when you're hungry, you feel tired, your brain seems to be in a fog and you're more irritable than usual? However, to get the most benefits from carbohydrates, make sure you select the right kind.

There are three types of carbohydrates:

→ Sugar: This simple form of carbohydrate can be found naturally in some foods, such as dairy, fruits and vegetables. Sugar can come in the form of lactose (milk sugar), fructose (fruit sugar) or sucrose (table sugar).

→ Starch: Complex carbohydrates like these are made up of bonded sugar. Vegetables, beans, peas and grain all contain starch.

→ Fiber: This is also a complex carbohydrate. Fiber can be found in vegetables, fruit, beans, peas and whole grains. Fiber helps keep your digestive system humming and keeps your blood cholesterol levels at healthy quantities.

Most carbohydrates can naturally be found in plant-based foods, such as the following:

→ Legumes

→ Fruit

→ Seeds

→ Vegetables

→ Grains

→ Nuts

Carbohydrates can also take the form of added sugar or starch that is added to food. This is usually added to processed food or recipes. This type of sugar has been linked to various diseases such as diabetes, heart disease and obesity (Satrazemis, 2018). Extra sugar is just that, nutrient-empty sugar. It adds empty calories to your food intake with no added nutritional benefits for your body.

Refined carbohydrates have been processed or have added sugar. They are less nourishing than their whole counterparts because the nutrients are stripped away. An example of a refined carb is white rice which has its germ, bran and husk removed. Those parts have vital nutrients.

When you consume carbohydrates, they are absorbed into your body as glucose. Glucose is also released in your bloodstream. Your cells absorb this simple sugar and when your blood sugar level goes down, your liver and muscles release stored sugar, called glycogen. The liver stores about 100 grams of glycogen. The glycogen in the liver can be released when needed to stabilize blood sugar levels. Meanwhile, muscles store around 500 grams of glycogen. However, it can only be used by muscle cells during long intervals of intense physical activity. When too many carbohydrates are eaten, the glycogen is then stored as fat. Therefore, when you consume more carbohydrates than you use, that is when you start gaining weight.

The more muscle mass you have, the more efficient your body is at storing glucose, instead of hoarding it as fat. This is one of the benefits of weight training and building your muscles.

When your body does not have enough glucose, your muscles can be broken down and converted into glucose to make sure your brain has enough energy to function. This is how your body survives in extreme conditions. It is definitely not an ideal or even safe scenario because you need your muscles for movement. Also, using protein instead of carbohydrates puts a lot of stress on your kidneys. Consuming enough carbohydrates makes sure this doesn't occur.

Benefits of Carbohydrates

Cutting out carbohydrates completely from your diet isn't healthy. You would be missing out on essential nutrients provided from eating whole grains and fruit, such as fatty acids, fiber, vitamins and minerals and phytonutrients. Without enough carbohydrates in your diet, you may experience dizziness, digestive problems and physical and mental weakness.

Consumption of foods high in fiber benefits your heart's health and your blood sugar levels. Soluble fiber helps absorb bile into your small intestine, preventing your body from reusing it. It also forces your liver to produce more bile by using cholesterol that would otherwise be in your blood.

While fiber is also a type of carbohydrate, it does not raise your blood sugar like other forms do. It even slows down the absorption of carbohydrates in your system, resulting in lower blood-sugar levels after meals. The Institute of Medicine recommends an intake of 14 grams of fiber per 1,000 calories (Szalay, 2017).

Eating foods high in fiber can also help you lose weight. These foods make you feel full faster and for a longer period, so you don't eat as much. Also, most food that is high in fiber tends to be low in calories.

Carbohydrates are important to your mental health. A study found that those on a low-carb, high-fat diet experienced more anger, anxiety and depression compared to those on a low-fat, high-carb diet. Scientists believe that carbohydrates may help in the production of serotonin, a chemical that contributes to feelings of happiness and well-being (Szalay, 2017).

Aside from carbs helping to keep you happy, it may also aid your memory. Tufts University did a study and put overweight women on a no-carb diet for one week. They tested their spatial memory, cognitive skills and visual attention. Afterwards, they discovered that those on the no-carb diet did worse on the tests than the women who were on a low-calorie diet, which had a healthy amount of carbs (Szalay, 2017).

Good carbohydrates, such as whole, unprocessed fruit and vegetables, and whole grains, are packed with nutrients such as polyunsaturated fats, micronutrients, antioxidants and fiber.

Consumption of sugar has a detrimental effect on our health over time. One way to determine a particular food's effect is through the glycemic index. This index ranks various carbohydrates from 0 to 100 of and gauges its potential to raise your blood sugar after eating. The higher the food is on the glycemic index means a higher potential to raise your blood sugar. Food such as potatoes, white bread and foods that contain white flour are on the higher end of the spectrum. Whole grains, vegetables and beans, on the other hand, fall on the lower end of the glycemic index. Eating food that has fat and protein along with those with simple sugars helps in slowing down digestion. That, in turn, doesn't cause a spike in your blood sugar, compared to consuming foods high in simple sugar on its own.

Consistent spikes in your blood sugar over a long period leads to pre-diabetes and insulin resistance.

Carbohydrates should make up 45 to 65 percent of the calories you consume daily (Government Publishing Office, 2011). One gram of carbohydrates equal to four calories (*Carbohydrates 101: The Benefits of Carbohydrates* , n.d.). So if you were to go on a 2,000-calorie diet, carbohydrates should make up 900 to 1,300 calories of the food you consume. That's 225 to 325 grams of carbohydrates. People who do high-intensity exercise and those who have more muscle mass can eat higher amounts of carbohydrates to keep their energy up. Those who develop type 2 diabetes, are obese, or have metabolic syndrome would do well to lower their carbohydrate intake to keep themselves healthy. The recommended dietary allowance for carbohydrates is at least 130 grams for adults per day, and at least 25 grams of fiber daily for women, 38 grams of fiber for men.

Packaged foods normally lists the number of carbohydrates they contain on the label.

What do carbohydrates do?

→ Provide energy. Carbohydrates are always the first source of energy your body burns. Once consumed, your body breaks down complex sugars into simple sugars and absorbed into your bloodstream, then known as blood sugar or blood glucose. With the help of insulin, the sugar enters your cells and provides energy. Any extra sugar goes to your muscles, liver, or other cells, or is converted to fat.

→ Lowers the chances of some diseases. A diet high in fiber reduces your risk of heart disease and type 2 diabetes. Fiber also keeps your digestive tract healthy and prevents constipation.

→ Helps you lose weight. Eating food packed with fiber helps you feel full faster and for a longer time with fewer calories.

What Carbohydrates to Eat

Focus on eating quality carbohydrates. Good carbohydrates are the ones that are high in fiber and take longer to break down into simple sugar. Here are characteristics of good foods:

→ Nutritionally dense. Fresh fruits and vegetables are high in nutrients.

→ High fiber. Carbs that are high in fiber to make you full faster and longer. Keep in mind that meat, dairy and sugar do not have fiber and "white" foods (refined foods such as white bread, white rice, etc.) have had all or most of their fiber removed during processing. The more unprocessed and natural the food is, the higher the fiber content it has. Food such as whole grains, vegetables, oatmeal, beans, nuts, legumes and fruit are all high in fiber. Look at the ingredients listed on the packaging. If whole grain is listed as the first ingredient, that food is high in fiber. You may also check the nutrition facts on the label. If there are three to five grams of fiber listed, that food is high in fiber (Petersen, 2017).

→ Have low or moderate calorie versions. Dairy products are a good source of protein and calcium, but opt for the low-fat options since the ones with higher fat also have higher calories. One gram of fat has nine calories. Some dairy products also have added sugar, so avoid those.

→ Absence of refined sugar or grains. Steer away from food that has added sugar and refined starches.

→ Low in sodium and saturated fat.

→ Low or no levels of cholesterol or trans fats.

Bad carbohydrates, in contrast, can be characterized as:

→ High in calories, but low in nutrients. This is also known as food with empty calories.

→ High in refined sugar and grains.

→ Low in fiber.

→ High in sodium, saturated fat, cholesterol or trans fats.

What Are "Added" Sugars?

The Dietary Guidelines for Americans recommend limiting the intake of added sugars to just 10% of your daily caloric intake (Baer, 2018). Try to avoid or lower consumption of food that have the following ingredients listed, as these are all added sugar:

→ Syrup

→ Brown sugar

→ Sucrose

→ Corn sweetener

→ Sugar

→ Corn syrup

→ Raw sugar

→ Dextrose

→ Molasses

→ Fruit juice concentrate

→ Malt syrup

→ Fructose

→ Maltose

→ High-fructose corn syrup

→ Invert sugar

→ Honey

→ Lactose

Cutting down or eliminating added sugars to your diet has proven to boost mood and energy levels and cut down on visceral fat (also known as belly fat). Visceral fat is the most dangerous type of fat as it is found near the intestines, liver and stomach and also in your arteries. It increases your chances of developing several life-threatening conditions such as type 2 diabetes, Alzheimer's disease, stroke and colorectal cancer, to name a few.

Carbo-Myths

Consuming Carbs Will Make You Gain Weight.
Overconsumption of any type of food, not just carbs, will cause you to gain weight. As mentioned earlier, eating food that is high in fiber could actually even help you to lose weight since fiber helps make you feel full faster. Also, your body works harder at digesting whole foods, so your body is burning more calories in that process than those made of simple carbs.

Fruits Aren't Healthy Because They Are High in Sugar.
While fruit does contain simple sugars, it also contains a lot of fiber, vitamins and minerals, all of which are very good for your health. Fruit comes with natural sugar, compared to added sugar which just has empty calories and contributes to weight gain and an increase in your risk of chronic diseases. Stick to eating whole fruit

instead of drinking fruit juice. Whole fruit has all the fiber in it, while fruit juice more often than not has added sugar.

Do Not Eat Carbohydrates at Night.

Carbohydrates in your body are processed the same way, no matter what time of the day it is. A study published in the American Journal of Clinical Nutrition showed that eating carbohydrates with a high glycemic index (GI) four hours before bedtime helps you fall asleep faster. This is possibly due to an increase of serotonin and tryptophan, brain chemicals that help you sleep (Miranda Hitti, n.d.).

Low Carb Diets Are the Most Effective Way to Lose Weight.

Weight loss from restricting carbs arises from a deficit in calorie consumption and from losing water weight, not from not eating carbs. It's not the carbs that are the problem, it's the type of carbs. Low carb diets are difficult to sustain in the long run, causing your body to crave the macronutrient, making you more likely to slip up and overindulge in unhealthy eating. Once you start devouring carbs again, you will most likely gain the weight back. Continually consuming healthy carbs will prevent your body from craving the unhealthy kind. Remember, your brain can only use glucose for energy. Not munching on enough carbs is bad for this vital organ that helps you make good decisions.

Basing the GI Level of a Carbohydrate on How Healthy It Is.

While it is important to look at the glycemic index of carbohydrates, especially those who are diabetic or experiencing insulin resistance, it should be considered as a whole. The GI does not paint the entire picture on how a certain food will impact your blood sugar. For example, if a high-glycemic-index food is eaten with protein, the protein can slow down digestion and absorption of the sugar into your bloodstream. Just using the GI without taking into account what other macronutrients are being consumed, how much of the carbohydrate is on your plate and what other nutrients the carbohydrate provides is inadequate.

Eating Carbs Will Make You Feel Sluggish Afterwards.

A study found that it is actually the size of the meal and the salt and protein content that makes you slip into a "food coma." Sugar had nothing to do with it (Forster, 2017).

Don't Eat Carbs Before Working Out.

When working out, your body needs the boost of energy that carbs can provide. It has to be the right type of carbohydrate though and consumed at the right time. Your cells need time to digest and convert the food into energy so give them an hour or two.

Protein Intake Is More Important Than Carbs.

While protein is important to be healthy, all macronutrients are important for your body, as they take on various roles in keeping your body functioning. In fact, some research shows that plant-based diets that are high in fiber and low in glycemic load are good for glucose metabolism (Dennett, 2016). It also determined that diets high in meat increase the risk of type 2 diabetes, plus some cancers such as lung, liver, and bowel cancer (*Protein and Diabetes*, 2019).

White Carbohydrates Are Unhealthy.

While white bread, rice, and flour have most of their nutrients stripped away during processing, other "white" carbohydrates that are healthy. Cauliflower, garlic and mushrooms are high in nutrients, for example. What to keep in mind here is not the color of the food, but if it has been processed.

CHAPTER 2: BASICS OF CARB CYCLING

What Is Carb Cycling?

Carb cycling is a diet method that requires you to alternate the number of carbohydrates you consume in a specified period to optimize intake. This method tries to match the level of carbohydrates you need, depending on your activity level. This methodology was frequently practiced by athletes and bodybuilders, but now is being practiced by non-athletes. Some of the advantages of carb cycling are as follows:

→ Increased energy: Your body is made to burn carbohydrates as its primary source of energy and can store up enough glycogen for up to two hours of exercise. Without depriving your body of this important macronutrient, your body doesn't have to go through any periods of adjustment where energy is depleted and it has to find other sources.

→ Long-term adherence to the diet: Because you don't deprive yourself of any type of macronutrient, your body won't crave it, helping you stick to it in the long run.

→ Improved cholesterol levels

→ Weight loss

→ Increased fat burning

→ Better balanced hormones

→ Better insulin sensitivity

→ Build-up of muscle tissue

Each year, 45 million Americans go on diets and spend $33 billion on weight-loss products. However, nearly two out of three Americans are overweight (*Weight Management*, 2017). Most diets aren't sustainable because they restrict you from eating certain types of food. The carb cycling diet doesn't do that as it allows for different levels of carbohydrates consumption depending on your level of activity.

Those who want to still perform well during physical activity, to lose weight or to conquer the dreaded weight-loss plateau will do well to go on the carb cycling diet. The idea is to increase carbohydrate intake on days when you need it and eliminate it on days you don't. How many carbohydrates you should have in a period depends on the following:

→ Shaping your physique: When you want to shed a few pounds, you can lower your carbohydrate intake. When you get to the stage where you work out and need energy, you can increase your carbohydrate intake.

→ Days you work out versus rest days: Carbohydrate intake is increased on days you work out and lowered on rest days.

→ Refeed days: These are scheduled days on your diet where you consume excessive but calculated amounts of carbohydrates to give your body a break from prolonged dieting. This is different from a cheat day, which is often unplanned and poorly calculated.

→ A planned increase in activity for the day: If you have a sport to play, a marathon to run or a planned hike that day, for example, you would increase your carbohydrate intake for the day.

→ Level of activity: More intense workouts warrant an increase in carbohydrate intake compared to lower intensity workouts. For lower intensity workouts, fat can provide more energy, but carbs can provide more energy for higher intensity workouts. Because fat takes longer to burn than carbohydrates, you have a ready source of energy for your body. This phenomenon is known as the crossover effect (Mawer, 2017).

→ Level of body fat: The higher body fat level you have, the lower your carbohydrate intake should be. This increases as you shed more pounds.

Normally, the carb cycling diet consists of three low carb intake days, two moderate carb intake days then two high carb intake days. The amount of protein consumed is typically the same on each day, but, depending on the program you follow, fat intake may inversely change depending on the number of carbohydrates consumed. However, the intake is different for each person, depending on the factors stated above. There will be a period of trial and error involved as you discover for yourself the right level of carbohydrate intake depending on your activity level, your goals and your lifestyle.

Increasing your carbohydrate intake during intense levels of activity helps replace muscle glycogen. Glycogen stores carbohydrates in our skeletal muscles and liver. It is the main energy source that is used during physical activity. Once glycogen is depleted in the muscles, fatigue sets in as the muscles break down. Having sufficient levels of glycogen allows you to exercise at a higher intensity for a longer period without feeling tired. That extra push you get from carbohydrates could mean you work out longer and harder, burning more calories. Carbohydrates also help your body recover faster from intense workouts by providing you with consistent energy. This is why it is important to eat carbohydrates before and after exercise – to give you the boost of energy you need when working out and to help your muscles recover and restore your energy after the workout.

Some believe that consuming carbohydrates after working out increases insulin production and encourages fat storage. However, carbohydrate intake after a workout promotes muscle regeneration, which helps you burn more calories, as insulin promotes both regenerations of muscles and protein synthesis. Of course, you need to stick to good carbohydrates for your post-workout food. Nicole Lana Lee, from One Green Planet, recommends the following (Lee, 2013):

→ Dark green vegetables

→ Banana

→ Chia seeds

→ Sweet potato

→ Apples

→ Brown rice

A higher level of carbohydrate intake improves leptin and ghrelin function. These hormones help regulate your weight and appetite.

Lower carbohydrate intake, on the other hand, forces your body to use stored fat as your energy source. Doing this frequently improves your body's ability to burn fat as fuel and improve metabolic flexibility, your body's ability to respond to fluctuations in metabolic needs.

Carb cycling also improves insulin sensitivity. A higher sensitivity means your cells are more effective in using blood glucose, subsequently lowering your blood sugar.

Carb cycling is beneficial for those who participate in sports or go through intensive workout sessions. This diet provides you with the right amount of carbohydrates for your energy needs, helping you improve performance.

Consuming fewer carbohydrates helps people lose weight and lower blood pressure, blood sugar and triglycerides. Low carb diets also raise good cholesterol levels and improve bad cholesterol readings. Compared to diets that restrict calories or fat, dieters are more successful at losing weight when going on a low carb diet.

Studies have shown that consuming lower amounts of carbohydrates leads to reducing belly fat. Having high levels of visceral fat (aka belly fat) is one of the characteristics of metabolic syndrome. It is one in a group of five conditions that increase your chances of suffering from a stroke, type 2 diabetes, or heart disease.

Prolonged deprivation of carbohydrates can be detrimental to your health and have negative effects on your metabolism. Eating too few carbs can harm your memory and brain functions since your brain's preferred source of energy comes from carbs. Also, low-carb diets put people at a higher risk of depression since serotonin levels become affected when you have low energy.

Carb cycling helps prevent this damage to your system by letting your body have the number of carbohydrates it needs.

Carb Cycling for Women

Is the carb cycling diet beneficial for women? Yes, it absolutely is. Women tend to accumulate more fat than men, especially about their waists and hips. The cycle of low carb and high carb intake helps burn stored fat and increases your metabolism.

With the keto and low-carb diets, women struggle with the balance in their hormone levels. Between the fluctuations related to menstruation and menopause, there are enough ups and downs with your hormones already without having your food habits bounce them around as well.

Consuming higher levels of carbohydrates means there is a need for more insulin in your body. Insulin tells your kidneys to retain sodium which, in turn, causes water retention. This is normally a problem for women, particularly when they are about to get their periods. Carb cycling helps reduce water retention. During periods of low carb intake, you reduce the insulin in your body which in turn signals for your kidneys to lose excess water.

When you restrict your carbohydrate intake, your body may respond with an increase in cortisol, lower metabolism, an impacted hormone system and decreased thyroid output. It might also be harder to lose weight or even find the energy to exercise or move. However, with a cycle of low carb and high carb diet, leptin—a hormone that impacts energy—may get an improved response and keep your hormones better balanced.

Who Shouldn't Be on a Carb Cycling Diet

Those who are pregnant or breastfeeding should not try to live on the carb cycling diet. Opt for a balanced diet instead. Those who are underweight should also avoid this diet.

Avoid this diet also if you have kidney issues or an eating disorder. Constant counting of calories and carbohydrates might aggravate or trigger any eating disorders you may have and make you even more unhealthy.

You shouldn't follow the carb cycling diet if you're mood is severely affected by limiting carbohydrates or if you're constantly craving for carbohydrates. You might not be able to make the commitment if you experience guilt when allowing yourself to eat carbs. Past diets may have changed how you interact with food so you should address those issues before engaging in this type of plan.

Constantly feeling tired while on the diet should also be an indication this is not the approach for you. If you find this happens to you, take a break and re-assess why you feel this way.

Did you find the information on carb cycling helpful and informative? Write a review on Amazon. We would love to hear about it.

CHAPTER 3: CARB CYCLING VS OTHER DIETS

Ketogenic Diet

The ketogenic diet, or keto for short, originated as a way that would help treat those with epilepsy. It is a low-carb, high-fat diet, that not only helps you lose weight, but helps improve your health in other ways as well. It provides benefits from a variety of healthy conditions relating to insulin-related, metabolic, and neurological diseases, such as type 2 diabetes and prediabetes, acne, heart disease, brain injuries, cancer, and more. On the keto diet, you get most of your calories from fat, some from protein and very few from carbohydrates – no more than 50 grams per day. It is similar to the Atkins diet and other low-carb diets.

There are various types of keto diets:

→ Standard ketogenic diet: The most researched diet divides your daily caloric intake into 75 percent fat, 20 percent protein and 5 percent carbs.

→ High-protein ketogenic diet: Similar to the one above, this version has more protein. Your daily caloric intake consists of 60 percent fat, 35 percent protein and 5 percent carbs.

→ Cyclical ketogenic diet: This adaptation has you on the ketogenic diet for several days, followed by a day or two of carbohydrate refeeds.

→ Targeted ketogenic diet: This diet allows for carbs before and after working out.

By limiting carbohydrate intake, you force your body into a state of ketosis. If you do not have sufficient carbohydrates in your diet, your body turns to fat to supply energy. When it does, ketones are produced and lead to ketosis. When this process is achieved, your body starts becoming more efficient in burning fat as energy. The liver also turns fat into ketones to be used by your brain for energy. A study found that those who were on the ketogenic diet lost 2.2 times more weight than those on a low-fat, calorie-restricted diet. It also showed that the levels of HDL cholesterol and triglycerides improved. Another study showed that people on the keto diet lost three times more weight than those on the balanced diet that Diabetes UK recommends. Results also show that the keto diet improves insulin sensitivity by 75 percent and lowers blood sugar levels (Mawer, 2018).

If you're on the ketogenic diet, you will need to eliminate the following food from your diet to achieve ketosis:

→ Foods high in sugar: Candy, soda, ice cream, juices, cake, smoothies, etc.

→ Starchy food or grains: Cereal, wheat-based food, pasta, rice, etc.

→ Fruit: Only a small number of berries and tomatoes are permitted.

→ Legumes and beans: Chickpeas. peas, lentils, kidney beans, etc.

→ Tubers and root vegetables: Parsnips, potatoes, carrots, sweet potatoes, jicama, etc.

→ Diet, sugar-free, or low-fat products: Food marketed as diet or low-fat often replaces the fat with sugar to give it flavor, so not only are they high in simple carbohydrates, they are also highly processed. Even those labeled as sugar-free should be avoided as they are high in sugar alcohols and are highly processed.

→ Most sauces and condiments: Add-ons such as ketchup, mustard, barbecue sauce, mayonnaise, etc., normally contain added sugar and unhealthy forms of fat.

→ Food with unhealthy fats: Saturated and artificial trans fats are considered as unhealthy components that cause an increase in the risk of diet-based chronic diseases, weight gain and clogged arteries. Examples of these would be partially hydrogenated or hydrogenated vegetable oil, packaged snack foods such as chips and crackers, and commercially baked goods such as pizza dough, cakes and cookies.

→ Alcoholic beverages: These drinks have high-carbohydrate content.

You are encouraged to eat food from these groups, rotating among the different meats and vegetables to give your body a variety of nutrients:

→ Meat: Turkey and chicken, beef, pork, processed meats including bacon, sausage, and ham.

→ Fatty fish: Mackerel, salmon, tuna and trout.

→ Eggs: Whole eggs with omega-3 or pastured versions are best suited to this plan.

→ Cream and butter: Preferably from grass-fed cows.

→ Unprocessed cheeses: Mozzarella, cheddar, blue, cream or goat

→ Seeds and nuts: Chia seeds, almonds, pumpkin seeds, walnuts, flax seeds, etc.

→ Healthy oils: Avocado oil, extra virgin olive oil, coconut oil.

→ Avocados and freshly-made guacamole (not store-bought because this may contain added sugars and may be processed).

→ Low-carbohydrate vegetables: Peppers, green leafy vegetables, onions

→ Spices: Salt, pepper, herbs

It's easier also being on the ketogenic diet and eating out at restaurants since you don't need to keep a strict count of your macros. You just need to keep in mind what food you can and can't eat; stick to proteins and exchange carbohydrates with low-carb vegetables.

Those who go on a keto diet normally experience the "keto flu" lasting from a few days to about two weeks. This is due to the body adjusting from burning carbohydrates for energy to burning fat. During this period, dieters may experience:

→ Body aches and pains
→ Insomnia
→ Adrenal issues
→ Irritability
→ Hormone imbalance
→ Muscle soreness
→ Dry eyes
→ Nausea
→ Dizziness
→ Poor focus, confusion and brain fog
→ Stomach pains
→ Sore throat
→ Cravings for sugar
→ Chills
→ Headache
→ Constipation

The ketogenic diet may also change the mineral and water balance in your body. It is recommended that you compensate by taking supplements such as magnesium, potassium and sodium, plus add extra salt to your food.

The ketogenic diet will not let you build muscles as efficiently, compared to a diet with a moderate amount of carb consumption. Therefore, it is not suitable for athletes or for people who want to put on muscle. If you're eating more fat than protein, you may lose weight, but it could be muscle that you're losing. With less muscle mass, your metabolism decreases. When you go off the ketogenic diet and regain much of the weight back, it comes back as fat, not muscle. You will be at the same starting weight as when you started the diet, but with less muscle, making it more difficult to lose weight again. Being on a keto diet may also prevent you from performing at your best physically because your body is in a more acidic state.

Due to the lack of fiber in your diet, you may get diarrhea while on the keto diet. This may also be due to your gallbladder getting overwhelmed from the high levels of fat you're consuming or food items you might be eating more of while on this diet, such as dairy or artificial sweeteners.

If you have diabetes, much like with any change in your lifestyle, you should consult with your doctor first before going on the keto diet. And if you do get the green light to go on this diet, you should check your blood sugar several times a day. For diabetics, being in a state of ketosis might trigger ketoacidosis. This process happens when your body stores too many ketones and the blood becomes too acidic. Acidic blood can damage the brain, kidneys and liver. If it goes untreated, it may cause death. Symptoms of ketoacidosis include difficulty breathing, dry mouth, bad breath, frequent urination and nausea.

Health experts say the keto diet isn't healthy or sustainable for the long term, due to it being so restrictive. Josh Axe, a clinical nutritionist, suggests that you shouldn't stay on the keto diet for longer than 90 days, and to find a more sustainable diet after. One of the main problems of being on the keto diet is most people gain the weight back once they reintroduce carbohydrates into their diets. The resulting weight fluctuations may contribute to an eating disorder or an unhealthy relationship with food. Most people who go on the keto diet have a problem with portion control and binge eating. Restricting carbohydrates will not get to the root cause of those issues. A counselor or lifestyle coach to help you get to the bottom of your food issues better.

Those who opt to go on the keto diet without the guidance of their doctors or nutritionists may end up having poor nutrition. This could raise their cholesterol levels and increase the risk of diabetes.

A study presented at the European Society of Cardiology Congress showed a possible link between those who follow very low-carb diets and the highest risk of dying from cardiovascular diseases, cancer and other chronic diseases. Another study published in the Lancet suggested that people who are on a low-carb high-animal-protein diet have a higher risk of early death compared to those who ate carbs in moderation (MacMillan, 2019).

Our bodies are meant to burn carbohydrates and do so more efficiently, compared to other macronutrients. Our bodies burn only 3 percent of fat through the process of conversion and storage, compared with 23 percent of carbohydrates burned through the same process.

Also, carbohydrates have fewer calories compared to fat on a gram-per-gram comparison, meaning you can eat more carbohydrates and still maintain a caloric deficit, than when you go on a high-fat diet. As mentioned before, weight loss is about having a deficit in the overall calories consumed.

You can combine the keto diet and carb cycling diet to gain the keto diet benefits of increased focus and energy, fat burning, and decreased appetite, but at the same time providing your body with carbohydrates it needs to function properly. You can do this by going very low carb or no-carb/high fat six days out of the week, then on the seventh day, refeed with about 150 grams of carbs. You will not be in ketosis on that day, but your body will return to ketosis once it burns through all the carbs you've consumed that day.

By cycling carbs, you are not yoyo dieting, which is demoralizing and not supportive of your overall health. Rather than gaining and losing weight over and over again, you can find a way to give your body what it needs, like dropping pounds consistently instead of quickly.

Volumetrics Diet

Developed by Dr. Barbara Rolls, a nutrition professor from Penn State University, this diet is meant to develop healthy eating habits rather than restrictive ones. The idea is to focus on consuming foods that are lower in calories but high in nutrients and water content – low-energy dense and high-nutrient dense. These are foods like low-fat dairy, whole grains, vegetables and fruit. These types of food improve appetite control and help in overall weight loss. Some studies show that food that is high in energy contributes to women developing a higher risk of type 2 diabetes and breast cancer (Radigan et al., 2019).

This diet doesn't restrict you from eating anything and acknowledges that all macronutrients are essential for a healthy body. This approach makes this diet easier to sustain because you get less cravings since you're allowed to eat all types of food. By focusing on eating low-calorie foods, you can eat as much as you like and not feel depressed, fatigued or hungry, traits which normally come with most diets.

Food is grouped into four categories, depending on how energy-dense they are:

Group 1 : This includes broth-based soups, non-starchy vegetables and fruit, and non-fat milk.

Group 2 : This includes low-fat dishes, starchy vegetables and fruit, legumes, grains, low-fat meat, and breakfast cereal.

Group 3 : This includes cake, meat with higher fat content, ice cream, cheese, pretzels, pizza, bread, salad dressing and French fries.

Group 4 : This includes oil, crackers, butter, chips, nuts, cookies and chocolate.

Group 1 has the least energy-dense food, and as you move towards Group 4, the food becomes more energy-dense. Food from Group 1 is considered as "free" food you can consume any time, while food from the other groups requires portion control to manage your calorie intake.

Aside from the food, the Volumetrics diet has a plan for working to get up to 30 minutes of exercise each day for most days of the week.

This diet plan is well-researched and approaches weight loss healthily. It stresses the importance of a balanced diet consisting of whole grains, fruits, and vegetables, instead of eliminating certain foods from your diet. It also focuses on what you can eat instead of what you are deprived of. It comes with recipes for you to follow. Since the diet is flexible, you can easily modify and replace ingredients, based on your tastes.

The diet is well balanced but you may not see weight loss immediately. It is not a quick-fix diet but more of a way to change your lifestyle to become healthier in the long run.

What may be off-putting is the emphasis on home-cooked meals and calculating the energy density of the food you're consuming. Also, Dr. Rolls recommends keeping a record of what you eat and how much physical activity you do, which may be too cumbersome for some people.

Eating low-calorie food that is high in water may not keep you full too long, compared to eating nutrient-dense food.

The volumetrics diet may not work for dieters who seek rigid rules on what they can and cannot eat. Some people prefer more clear guidelines to keep them on track.

Intermittent Fasting

Fasting is an ancient tradition practiced by many cultures around the world. Intermittent fasting claims to facilitate weight loss, improve your metabolism and even prolong your life. There are different methods of intermittent fasting:

→ 16/8 Method: This method allows you to eat within an eight-hour window, and fast for the rest of the 16 hours in the day. Water, coffee and other zero-calorie beverages are allowed to be consumed throughout the day. Women are recommended to fast for only 14 to 15 hours though, because they seem to do better with slightly shorter fast periods. Like other diets, the quality and quantity of food you eat during the eight-hour window are important. The diet will not work if you overeat or eat a lot of junk food. You may repeat the cycle as often as you like – for example, two or three times out of the week, or daily. The 16/8 method is the most popular technique practiced by those new to intermittent fasting as this requires them to just skip breakfast and have lunch as their first meal of the day then dinner within a span of 8 hours.

→ The 5:2 Method: This method allows you to eat normally five days out of the week, and restrict your calorie intake to 500 to 600 calories two days out of the week.

→ Eat Stop Eat Method: This method allows you to eat normally for one to two days, then change to a 24-hour fast for one day, then eat normally again for another one to two days after that. Similar to the 16/8 method, water, coffee, tea and other zero-calorie beverages are allowed throughout the fast, but no solid food. During the "Eat" periods, you have to make sure to eat normally; do not overeat, as this will reverse any calorie deficit you gain during fasting days. Doing a 24-hour straight fast seems daunting at first, so if you choose this method, you may start with a 14- to 16-hour fast first, then work your way up to 24 hours.

→ Alternate Day Fasting: This method allows you to eat normally for 24 hours and then fast for 24 hours. Some participants eat a maximum of 500 calories on fasting days, while others only consume water, coffee, tea and other zero-calorie beverages.

→ Warrior Diet: The warrior diet allows you to eat small amounts of fruit and vegetables throughout the day and have one full heavy meal at night within a four-hour window. The types of fruit and vegetables you're allowed to eat are similar to those on the paleo diet – whole and unprocessed food.

→ Spontaneous Fasting: Spontaneous fasting is fasting whenever you don't feel like eating. It is not planned and can be done anytime you wish.

Intermittent fasting is simple to follow, compared to other diets that have a lot of strict rules. It can provide quick results without much effort on your end. It is flexible in terms of what you can and can't eat, as long as you keep food intake within the time you're supposed to be eating. Of course, to maximize the benefits of your fast, it is best not to overeat and to stick to low-energy, high-nutrient dense whole foods. Many believe that intermittent fasting helps you live longer, boost your brain function and improve your blood sugar levels.

Intermittent fasting is easier to sustain compared to other diets that heavily restrict or eliminate certain food groups.

However, intermittent fasting can also cause some to overeat during the time they are allowed to eat, to compensate for the fast. This may lead to the development of unhealthy eating habits, digestive problems and weight gain. The possibility of developing unhealthy eating habits is a reason why this diet is not recommended for those with eating disorders.

At the beginning of the fast, you may feel tired, weak and hungry. Once your body adjusts and gets used to fasting, these side effects should disappear. Also, try to increase your protein intake at the end of your caloric intake period to keep you full longer. Some people though may not do well with fasting no matter what they do. If this is the case for you, don't force it, and look for an alternative diet better suited for you.

Other side effects some people experience while intermittent fasting is brain fog and tiredness, due to skipping breakfast. Eating breakfast normally gives you a boost of energy to keep you alert during the day. If breakfast is what you need in your life, pay attention to your body, and adjust your caloric intake period to include breakfast instead.

Intermittent fasting may also trigger eating disorders, instead of having a positive and healthy relationship with food. Binge eating is also a concern for those who go on this diet. Because of excessive hunger, you may end up overeating to compensate for the hours you fasted. If you tend to binge eat, it may be best to find a diet that will let you eat around the clock instead of within a short window.

Some people who do intermittent fasting experience trouble sleeping. Talk to a doctor or nutritionist to make sure you're not hurting your health. The same goes for constant mood changes you get while on the diet. You need to speak with your doctor or a nutritionist to figure out if there is a better fasting schedule to lessen the mood swings.

If you are diabetic, it is important to consult with your doctor first, if you plan on going on an intermittent fasting diet as it may make it more challenging for you to control your blood sugars. Some symptoms that may appear that could tell you there is something not right are dizziness, persistent nausea and headaches. Going on intermittent fasting as a diabetic puts you at risk of becoming hypoglycemic. If your doctor gives you the "go" signal to go on this diet, you must check your blood sugar levels several times a day to make sure they are still within safe levels.

Intermittent fasting may cause hair loss, due to a lack of proper nutrients such as B vitamins and proteins. Intermittent fasting doesn't restrict you in what type of food you can eat, but it may be more difficult to eat a balanced diet when you only have a few hours to eat. Evaluate the nutrition in what you eat during the caloric intake period to make sure you're not depriving yourself of crucial nutrients for your body. There is also a risk of dehydration when going on the intermittent fasting diet. While you are allowed to drink throughout the day, you're limiting water you normally get in food that you eat throughout the day to just the caloric intake period. You have to take the extra effort in keeping yourself hydrated throughout the day to avoid constipation.

Some believe intermittent fasting isn't as effective for women, compared to men. There are also studies done on animals that suggest intermittent fasting may affect reproduction and fertility in females (*Is Intermittent Fasting Safe for Fertility?*, 2020).

Sudden weight loss in women or in prolonged instances where they do not get the right amount of nutrition could have an effect on their menstrual cycles. It might slow it down or stop it completely so track your periods to see if you experience this effect.

Vegan Diet

Veganism is a way of life wherein you consciously exclude any form of animal cruelty and exploitation in your way of living, whether is it clothing, food or other consumer goods. Food that comes from animals is not allowed, along with food that is derived from animals, and those that have animal byproducts in them. People go on the vegan diet, not just to lose weight, but also for health, environmental and ethical reasons. A vegan diet prohibits any animal products such as dairy, eggs and meat. The diet only includes plants and food made from plants. Vegans tend to have lower body mass indexes (BMI) and are thinner than non-vegans. Vegans may consume fewer calories than non-vegans since most of the food on a vegan diet tends to be higher in fiber, resulting in weight loss.

To be healthy while on the vegan diet:

→ Keep yourself hydrated and drink enough fluids every day (six to eight glasses).

→ Eat at least five servings of different fruits and vegetables daily.

→ Ingest limited portions of spreads and oils, sticking to the unsaturated kind.

→ Whenever possible, choose whole grain bread, rice and pasta.

→ Base your meals on starchy carbohydrates such as potatoes, rice or yams.

→ Make sure to always include beans and pulses in your meals so you have enough protein in your diet.

→ Include dairy alternatives in your diet such as soy yogurt and soy drinks. Make sure you choose the low-fat and low-sugar variations.

You may eat food that is high in salt, sugar or fat, but keep it to a small amount and sparingly.

There are different type of vegan diets (Petre, MS, RD (NL), 2016):

→ Whole-food: This diet consists of whole plant foods such as seeds and nuts, fruits, legumes, whole grains and vegetables.

→ Raw-food: This diet consists of raw seeds, nuts, vegetables, fruits and other plant foods cooked at a temperature no higher than 118°F.

→ 80/10/10: Also known as the fruitarian diet, this consists of 80 percent of your daily calorie intake from carbohydrates, 10 percent from protein, and 10 percent from fat. It is a low-fat, raw food vegan diet consisting mostly of leafy greens and raw fruit. The food must remain raw because cooking damages the nutrients in the food.

→ Starch solution: Similar to the 80/10/10n diet, but instead of fruit, its focus is on cooked starches such as corn, rice and potatoes. This diet is also low in fat and high in carbohydrates.

→ Raw till 4: A mashup of the 80/10/10 and starch solution diets, this diet consists of consuming raw food until 4 p.m. then switching to consuming a cooked vegan meal.

→ Thrive diet: Followers of this diet only eat raw or minimally cooked whole, plant-based food.

→ Junk food vegan diet: This is a diet that consists of heavily processed vegan foods such as vegan desserts, mock cheeses and meats and fries.

A vegan diet may help improve your blood sugar levels. Studies have shown that vegans are at up to a 78 percent lower risk of developing type 2 diabetes compared to non-vegans. They also have higher insulin sensitivity and lower blood sugar levels. For diabetic vegans, their diets can lower their blood sugar levels up to 2.4 times compared to other diets recommended by the National Cholesterol Education Program, American Dietetic Association and the American Heart Association (Petre, MS, RD (NL), 2016). This may be because, again, due to the higher fiber food that the diet includes, which stabilizes the blood sugar levels after eating. Also, weight loss from the diet leads to lower blood sugar levels.

Aside from improving blood sugar control, a vegan diet can also help make your heart healthier. The risk of developing high blood pressure is 75 percent lower and 42 percent lower from dying from heart disease on a vegan diet. Several studies have shown that vegan diets also reduce total cholesterol and low-density (also known as LDL or "bad") cholesterol compared to other diets (Petre, MS, RD (NL), 2016).

While further studies need to be made, there have been some observations showing benefits such as (Petre, MS, RD (NL), 2016):

→ Lower risk of developing cancer by 15 percent

→ Reduced symptoms of arthritis such as morning stiffness, joint swelling and pain.

→ Better kidney function for diabetics

→ A lower risk of developing Alzheimer's disease

While a vegan diet, when done right, can result in weight loss and better control of your blood sugar, there is a risk of nutritional deficiencies with your diet. That is why some level of planning is also involved while on this diet to ensure you're getting the complete required nutrients daily. Vegans are usually deficient in zinc, vitamin B12, calcium, vitamin D, iron, iodine and long-chain omega-3s (Petre, MS, RD (NL), 2016). Substitutions for animal products are available and these are:

→ Vegetables and fruits: Leafy greens for example are high in calcium and iron.

→ Tofu, seitan and tempeh: These are high in protein and can replace eggs, meat, poultry and fish. Tofu also has calcium and omega-3 fatty acids.

→ Sprouted and fermented plant foods: These contain vitamin K2 and probiotics. They also help in mineral absorption.

→ Legumes and pulses: They are full of nutrients, such as calcium and iron. Walnuts also have omega-3 fatty acids.

→ Whole grains and cereals: These are an excellent source of complex carbohydrates, minerals, fiber, B-vitamins, vitamin D, and iron. Some, like quinoa and amaranth, are also high in protein.

→ Nuts and nut butters: These are high in vitamin E, iron, selenium, fiber, zinc and magnesium. Opt for the unroasted and unblanched varieties to get the maximum amount of nutrients.

→ Nutritional yeast: High in protein, this can be added to food. There are also nutritional yeasts that are B12-fortified.

→ Seeds: They provide protein and omega-3 fatty acids.

→ Algae: These provide protein and some varieties also contain iodine.

→ Plant milk and yogurts: Look for those fortified with calcium, and vitamins B12 and D.

→ Tahini and sesame seeds: They provide calcium

→ Dried fruit: Apricots, raisins, figs, and prunes deliver calcium and iron.

→ Sunlight: Exposure to the sun fuels your body with vitamin D.

→ Fortified fat spreads: These provide vitamin D

→ Vitamin D supplements: Check the label to make sure the vitamin D does not come from animals.

Should there still be a deficiency, you may turn to supplements to compensate for the deficit. Talk to your doctor to get the necessary tests done to make sure you're covering your body's nutritional needs while on the vegan diet, and discuss what nutritional supplements you need to make sure you stay healthy.

Going vegan requires a big adjustment on your part. For example, you will need to adjust your food consumption to make sure you're getting enough food each day. As animal-derived food has more calories than a plant-based food, you will need to eat more to make sure you're getting enough calories you need in a day. When starting your vegan diet, track your food consumption over the next few days to see if you're getting enough calories and sufficient macros from your diet.

You may also experience cravings for non-vegan food which is normal since that's what your body has been used to for a while. Take your time transitioning. Most people who go all-in so quickly aren't able to sustain it. If your body had been used to consuming food with animal products, added sugar and unhealthy chemicals, it will take some time for it to heal from the goodness of whole vegan foods.

At the start of a vegan diet, you may feel lethargic and tired. This might mean you're undereating or not eating nutritious food. Again, track what you eat over the next few days so you can see where you need to make adjustments.

Digestive issues may also pop up when you start a vegan diet. This is usually because your body is trying to get used to a different sort of food. If you're eating mostly whole vegan food, you're adding a lot of fiber to your diet, a lot more than what your gut might be used to. Again, it's best to transition slowly to give your digestive system time to adjust.

Be careful of vegan convenience foods as those usually have a lot of fat and sodium which can lead to water retention and weight gain. Also, avoid food that has added sugar or oil and those that are highly processed. Stick to whole vegan foods and make sure you eat more than what you normally did pre-veganism to make sure you get enough calories in a day. Keep in mind that just because something is labeled vegan, doesn't mean it's healthy and won't put you at risk for diet-induced chronic diseases. French fries and Oreo cookies meet the vegan criteria, but clearly are not healthy. Convenience vegan food should not be habitually consumed if you want to maintain a healthy diet.

Being a new vegan also means trying to cook new dishes with ingredients you might possibly have not had before. Subtract animal products from your diet gradually, replacing them with vegan alternatives. This will ensure you're getting the same nutrients as before. Buy a vegan cookbook so you can explore new dishes and new cooking techniques.

Vegans run the risk of not consuming enough calories and important nutrients from cutting out meat and animal products from their diet. Some of these nutrient deficiencies are quite serious, such as a vitamin B12 deficiency, which can cause neurological effects such as issues with balance, numbness in the hands and feet and even irreversible dementia. Other health problems could be fatigue, a weaker immune system, rashes, a higher risk of bone fractures from not consuming enough calcium and vitamin D, and high blood pressure.

Many vegans also experience iron deficiency. Iron is vital for your body because it helps in transporting oxygen throughout your body. There are two types of iron – non-heme iron and heme iron. Heme iron comes from animal products. Vegans rely on non-heme iron, however, it is not as readily absorbed by your body compared to the heme variation. Not getting enough iron can make you anemic, which is a serious condition, that occurs when your body doesn't produce enough red blood cells.

Getting sufficient protein in your diet may also be another challenge, but bear in mind that there are plenty of plant-based foods that can provide protein. Protein deficiencies can cause swelling, fatigue and hair loss so watch for those signs.

CHAPTER 4: CARB CYCLING, INSULIN RESISTANCE AND DIABETES

Insulin Resistance

Insulin resistance occurs when your body doesn't respond to this hormone the way it is supposed to. When the cells in your liver, body fat and muscles ignore the signal insulin is sending out, they don't collect the glucose in the bloodstream and store it in the cells. If there's constantly too much sugar in your blood, your cells adapt to the new sugar levels; they don't respond to the normal amount of insulin your body releases and don't absorb as much of the sugar.

This can lead to premature aging, prediabetes, type 2 diabetes, gestational diabetes, obesity and inflammatory age-related diseases.

Because of the damage high blood sugar wreaks on your cells, the risk of getting a stroke or heart attack doubles, and triples the chances that the attack will be deadly. Your risk of developing Alzheimer's and dementia also increases. High insulin levels promote the growth of tumors and subdue your body's ability to protect itself by killing malignant cells, which means your chances of developing cancers of the uterus, bladder, prostate, breast, pancreas, cervix and colon are higher.

Your ethnicity, age and genetics affect insulin sensitivity but the main culprits are all controllable factors such as getting enough sleep, being overweight or obese, smoking, carrying too much belly fat and not getting enough exercise. With insulin resistance, your body needs more of the hormone than usual to process the sugar in your bloodstream. Your body responds by producing more and more insulin and over time, your pancreas wears out and cannot keep up with the demand.

When this happens and you do not get adequate insulin, your blood sugar levels start rising and you could develop prediabetes or type 2 diabetes. Non-alcoholic fatty liver disease could also develop from insulin resistance and could increase your chances of developing heart disease and liver damage.

Symptoms of Insulin Resistance include:

→ Dark skin patches or acanthosis nigricans. If the insulin resistance is severe, you may start developing patches of dark skin on your armpits, the back of your neck, your knuckles, knees and elbows.

→ Having a waist that measures 35 inches or more if you're a woman; 40 or more if you're a man.

→ Developing signs of metabolic syndrome: If you have three or more of the following ailments or take medication for three or more of those ailments, you might have metabolic syndrome, which creates insulin resistance:
○ High fasting blood sugar, which could be an early sign of diabetes.
○ Blood sugar at 100 to 125 mg/dl or over 125
○ Blood pressure at 130/85 Hg or higher
○ Triglyceride levels of 150 or higher
○ Low high-density lipoprotein (HDL) levels or low-density lipoprotein (LDL) levels that are below 50 if you're a woman and 40 if you're a man.
Insulin resistance can be treated through the following:
→ Insulin injections and pumps.
→ Exercise and more sleep.
→ Keto and low carb diets.
→ Improving your body composition to be closer to the ideal – less than 12 percent body fat for men, less than 18 percent body fat for women, through interval cardio, circuit training, and strength training. At its peak performance, insulin will take the sugar in your body to your cells to use it as energy or to your liver and muscles to convert it to glycogen.
But of course, prevention is always better than the cure, so at first try some lifestyle changes instead of relying on medication to control your blood sugar.
To improve your insulin sensitivity and keep yourself healthy, make sure you do all three of the following:
→ Keep your weight at a healthy level
→ Exercise regularly
→ Get enough sleep

Type 2 Diabetes

With type 2 diabetes, your cells don't respond to insulin as efficiently and the glucose in your bloodstream builds up instead of getting stored in your cells. Chronic uncontrolled diabetes does a lot of damage to various organs and can lead to serious complications.
The early symptoms of type 2 diabetes are easy to dismiss because they are mild and not very extraordinary for the most part:
→ Blurry vision
→ Constant hunger

→ Itchy skin
→ Lethargy
→ Cottonmouth
→ Constant tiredness
→ Frequent thirst
→ Frequent urination
→ Weight loss

If you've had chronic high blood sugar, the symptoms of type 2 diabetes could also include:

→ Neuropathy or a feeling of numbness in your arms, legs, hands and feet.
→ Frequent yeast infections
→ Foot pain
→ Sores or cuts that don't seem to heal or take long to heal

The recommended daily allowance of carbohydrates for diabetics is the same for non-diabetics. However, diabetics should spread out the consumption of their carbohydrates to avoid their blood sugar from spiking. Limit your intake to 45 to 60 grams per meal or not more than 200 grams in a day (Carbohydrates 101: The Benefits of Carbohydrates, n.d.).

Many studies support a low-carb diet as beneficial for those with type 1 and 2 diabetes. In fact, before insulin was discovered, a low-carb diet was already the method being used to treat people with diabetes. Low-carb diets prevent your blood sugar from spiking, reducing the risk of complications from diabetes.

It is also recommended that diabetics consume complex carbohydrates and minimize, if not totally avoid, simple carbohydrates also to avoid their blood sugar spikes. The increase in insulin contributes to insulin resistance and makes it easier for your body to convert glucose into fat.

Aside from insulin resistance, consuming bad carbs elevates and drops your blood sugar faster, making you crave for your next meal sooner.

To determine the maximum amount of carbohydrates you can consume if diagnosed with type 2 diabetes, it is best to test your blood sugar before a meal and again one to two hours after eating to find your limit. Studies have shown that blood sugar levels improve when carbohydrate intake is between 20 to 90 grams per day, so you may opt to consume six, 10, or 25 grams of carbs per meal as long as your blood sugar remains below 140 mg/dl, which is the point when nerve damage occurs from excessive sugar in your blood (Spritzler & Marengo, 2020).

It is best to discuss with your doctor before making changes to your diet since your medication will need to be adjusted on low carb days of your carb cycle to prevent you from suffering from hypoglycemia.

Net Carbs

Only starchy and simple sugar carbohydrates can cause your blood sugar to increase. Fiber does not have that effect on your blood sugar since it doesn't break down into glucose. Sugar alcohols, such as sorbitol, maltitol, erythritol, and xylitol, are used to sweeten food marketed as "sugar-free."

To get your "net" carb content or the number of digestible carbs in your food, you can subtract the fiber and sugar alcohols your food contains. However, when it comes to sugar alcohols, some still cause an increase in blood sugar for those who have diabetes, so you need to be careful with this.

Also, take note that the Food and Drug Administration does not use "net carb" in its literature, but "total carbohydrates" instead.

The Glycemic Index

Here are some examples of some common food and their corresponding glycemic index (GI):

GI Range: ≤ 40 (Foods With Very Low GI):

→ Barley
→ Raw apples
→ Boiled carrots
→ Lentils
→ Cow's milk
→ Soybeans
→ Kidney beans

GI Range: 41-55 (Foods With Low GI):

→ Chocolate
→ Noodles and pasta
→ Sweet corn
→ Apple juice
→ Strawberry jam
→ Raw oranges/orange juice
→ Whole grain bread

→ Dates
→ Yogurt
→ Raw banana

GI Range: 56-70 (Foods With Intermediate GI):

→ Sourdough bread
→ Brown rice
→ Honey
→ Rolled oats
→ Pineapple
→ Soft drinks

GI Range >70 (Foods With High GI):

→ Rice crackers
→ White and wholemeal bread
→ White rice
→ Boiled potato
→ Mashed potatoes
→ Cornflakes
→ French fries

With the list above, you can assess more or less where in the spectrum your current diet is in terms of GI (The Functions of Carbohydrates in the Body : (EUFIC), 2012). Some studies link food with high GI levels to cause certain cancers, diabetes, heart disease and obesity (Szalay, 2017).

Several studies have shown that whole grains protect against type 2 diabetes and improves glucose metabolism and insulin sensitivity (Dennett, 2016).

As with any diet, it is best to consult with your doctor first before beginning.

CHAPTER 5: HOW TO GET STARTED ON THE CARB CYCLING DIET

The carb cycling diet requires a lot of planning, prepping and tracking in order to be successful. You need to count, measure and weigh your proteins, fats and carbohydrates. It's best for you to prepare your food at home, ahead of time, as it's easier to control and track the macros in your meal, than when getting takeout or eating out.

To get started, you need to track your macronutrients – mainly, your proteins, fats and carbohydrates. You can do this with an app on your phone or through a food journal.

How Many Carbohydrates Do You Need in One Day?

To start off, you need to determine how many calories you need in a day. As a general rule, to determine the number of calories to consume in a day, if you want to gain weight, multiply your body weight by 15. If you want to maintain your weight, multiply your body weight by 12. If you want to lose weight, multiply your body weight by 10. As with any diet, carb cycling will be effective for weight loss if there is a calorie deficit. To compute how many calories your required macronutrients will provide, keep in mind that carbohydrates and proteins each contribute four calories per gram. Fat has nine calories per gram.

As mentioned earlier, there is a lot of trial and error in figuring out how much carbohydrate you should ingest as it depends on a variety of factors such a sex, weight, age, level of activity and your overall health. As a starting point, for a high carbohydrate intake day, consume about 60 percent of your total calories from carbohydrates. And as a starting point for low carbohydrate intake, you can try 50 grams of carbohydrates in one day, which is the maximum amount of carbohydrates most people can have in order to reach ketosis. Ketosis is what happens when your body doesn't have enough carbohydrates to burn so it burns fat instead and produces ketones.

One option, instead of planning your carb intake daily, is planned per activity. For example, carbohydrates with sugar are eaten before and after intense workouts to provide your body with quick energy. The complex carbs are then saved for lower carbohydrate requirements so you can feel full faster and longer without eating so much.

There are also carbohydrate calculators online, such as on calculator.net that can help you figure out how much carbohydrate you should consume, depending on your fitness goals. Just keep in mind that this should just be a starting point and that you may adjust the carbohydrate levels later on as you see fit. If you don't lose any weight after the first week, you can try lowering your carbohydrate intake further. If you are dropping pounds, but find that you feel sluggish or have no energy, increase your carb intake a bit and see what effect it will have on your energy levels and weight.

Another way to calculate how many grams of carbohydrates you should have would be to base it on your weight. Get your weight in kilograms then multiply by the following, depending on your activity level:

→ Sedentary - lightly active: Your weight in kg x 2.5-3.5 grams

→ Moderately - heavily active: Your weight in kg x 3.5-4.5 grams

→ Extremely active: Your weight in kg x 5.0-7.0 grams

Match your high carb intake days on days where you will have high-intensity workouts. Keep your protein intake the same regardless of carbohydrate intake, but lower your fat intake when you increase your carbohydrate intake and vice versa.

Keeping Track of Your Macros

It is important to be meticulous in keeping track of your macros while carb cycling to ensure you have enough protein, fat and carbohydrates in your diet. There are apps available that you may download on your phone to help you keep track. Here are the five best apps to track your macros according to Men's Health Magazine (Matthews, 2019):

→ **MyPlate**: Answer a few questions and the app will provide you with a recommendation on how you can achieve your weight goals. You can keep track of your breakfast, lunch, dinner and snacks. The macros are broken down for each food listed and it will also show you a summary of your macro consumption for the day. This app is free to download for iOS and Android.

→ **My Fitness Pal**: This app has a large database of foods that lists the number of calories, macros and nutrients for each. The free version shows you a summary of your macro consumption for the day, while the paid version lets you set a goal for each macro. The app will provide a countdown as to how much more you can consume. You can also set your weight goals and input your exercise level. This app is free to download for iOS and Android.

→ **MyMacros+**: This also has a database of foods and their calories, macros and nutrient information. It can track your body weight and also has a macros countdown. For an additional fee, you can add its macro coach feature, which will tell you how many macros you need to achieve your goal. There is no free version and membership starts at $1.99 per month. It is available to download for both iOS and Android.

→ **LoseIt!**: The free version allows you to keep track of your meals and macros consumed. The premium version, which costs $29.99 per year, provides you with meal plans, shopping lists and exercise routines. This is available for iOS.

→ **Carb Manager**: This app also has a database of foods and also provides you with low-carb recipes. You may track your exercise, weight and body measurements with this app. Premium services are also available at $39.99 per year. This is available to download for both iOS and Android.

If you're old school and prefer to track using pen and paper, you may refer to the Denver's Diet Doctor to check the macros and calories for your food

What Should I Expect When Starting Carb Cycling?

Prepare yourself as your body adjusts to consuming low amounts of carbohydrates. You may feel the following for the first few days:

→ Mood swings

→ Insomnia

→ Bloating

→ Fatigue

→ Constipation

Make sure you are well-hydrated and replenish your body's electrolytes by eating bananas or drinking coconut water.

During your first few days of the diet, you may lose water weight - as much as five to 10 pounds. Losing weight slows down after the first week, but if you continue on the diet, you will still continue to lose fat.

CHAPTER 6: BEST FOODS FOR THE CARB CYCLING DIET

What Type of Carbohydrates Should You Eat?

The type of carbohydrates you consume also helps in maximizing intake. It's best to consume good carbohydrates that are high in fiber so you feel full longer. Good carbohydrates are those that are not processed and are digested slowly.

Types of good, complex carbohydrates are:

→ Whole grains: These grains contain bran, endosperm and germ. Consuming whole grains reduces the risk of diseases such as type 2 diabetes, heart disease, obesity and stroke.

→ Vegetables: Vegetables not only come with good carbohydrates, but also essential vitamins and minerals.

→ Fresh fruit: Like vegetables, fruit comes with good carbohydrates as well as vitamins and minerals. It is important to note the fruit should be fresh or unprocessed, as processed fruit usually has added sugar.

→ Legumes: These are high in fiber.

→ Tubers: These plant stems grow underground. Examples of tubers are potatoes, sweet potatoes and cassava. Tubers are a high source of vitamins and minerals, as well as antioxidants.

Most of the carbohydrates you consume should be from this list. They keep you full faster and for a longer period of time, compared to food with simple carbohydrates. Complex carbohydrates also take longer to digest, therefore keeping your blood sugar at a constant level instead of spiking.

High-Carb vs Low-Carb Food

For high-carb days, choose foods that are high in nutrients and slow-digesting. The following foods provide at least 12 grams of carbohydrates per serving:

→ Low-fat dairy products: low-fat milk or yogurt. There is an emphasis here on "low-fat" because food that is high in fat means it is higher in calories.

→ Whole grains: Emphasis on whole grain – grain that still has the bran, endosperm, and germ. These could be whole grain cereals and pasta, quinoa, oatmeal, amaranth, brown rice and barley.

→ Legumes: Soy beans, lentils, chickpeas, black beans, navy beans and pinto beans.

→ Fruit: Kiwi, berries, bananas, citrus fruits, pears, melons and apples. For fruit that has edible skin, you'll get more nutrients and fiber from eating the skin instead of peeling it off.

→ Starchy vegetables: Carrots, sweet potatoes, peas, yams and corn

→ Dark chocolate: Before anything, READ THE LABEL as the amount of carbohydrates varies per brand. On average, it should have 46 grams of carbohydrates per 100 grams of dark chocolate, or 13 grams of carbohydrates per ounce.

For low-carb days, focus on foods that provide no more than 10 grams of carbohydrates per serving, such as:

→ Soy milk and tofu

→ Non-starchy vegetables: Mushrooms, green leafy vegetables like spinach, lettuce, and cabbage, zucchini, asparagus, peppers, tomatoes, cucumbers, broccoli, green beans, and cauliflower.

→ Nuts and seeds: Pistachios, pumpkin seeds, peanuts, sunflower seeds, walnuts, almonds, and cashews.

→ Fruit: Most fruits are high in carbohydrates, but there are a few that are low carb such as strawberries, grapefruit, apricots, raspberries, lemons, kiwis, mulberries, and oranges.

What Type of Carbohydrates Should You Avoid?

Stay away from carbohydrates that are processed, low in fiber or have sugar or white flour. Cookies, white bread, cake, and cereal with high amounts of sugar in it are examples of carbohydrates you should be avoided. Go for spices to flavor your food instead of sauces as sauce usually contains added sugar.

Some plans recommend the carbohydrate you include based on the GI table, however, the GI table does not take into account how many grams of carbohydrates are in each specific food. Instead, assess carb quality on the glycemic load (GL), which takes into account the planned portion size along with the GI of the food (Satrazemis, 2018).

Keep an eye out for food marketed as "low fat." Fat in food makes it tasty. To keep it tasty while taking out fat, manufacturers add sugar and other fillers. Read the labels to truly understand what you are putting into your mouth.

If You Have Diabetes or Pre-Diabetes

If you're diabetic, it is best to stick to foods with low carbohydrate content, but are nutrient-dense.

Make sure you get enough protein in every meal. To boost your protein intake, you may eat enough of the following food until you feel full:

→ Cream cheese, olive oil, sour cream, cream and butter

→ Seafood, poultry and meat

→ Olives

→ Eggs

→ Avocados

→ Cheese

→ Non-starchy vegetables

You may eat the following foods in moderation. The quantity will depend on the amount of carbs your body can tolerate without causing your blood sugar to spike:

→ 4 ounces of dry white or red wine

→ 1.5 ounces of liquor

→ Maximum of 1 cup of berries

→ Maximum of 1 cup of plain, Greek yogurt

→ Maximum of 1 cup of squash such as hubbard, butternut, pumpkin, acorn or spaghetti

→ Maximum of ½ cup of cottage cheese

→ Maximum of 30 grams of dark chocolate that is at least 85 percent cocoa

→ Maximum of 2 ounces of peanuts and nuts

→ Maximum of 2 tbsp of chia seeds or flaxseeds

→ Maximum of ½ cup of legumes

A low carb diet will make you lose water weight during the first few days due to lower insulin levels causing your kidneys to release water and sodium. As not to lose too much sodium, you may add extra salt in your food, drink broth or eat salty, low carb foods such as olives to compensate. If you have high blood pressure, kidney disease or congestive heart failure, consult with your doctor first before adding more sodium to your diet.

Avoid the following food as these will cause your blood sugar to shoot up rapidly:

→ Ice cream, pastries and other baked goods, candy and desserts

→ Corn, bread, cereal, pasta and other grains, especially white bread, white pasta and white rice. These are processed foods that contain very little fiber and a high amount of simple sugars. Sweetened cereal is also one of the worst ways to start the day if you are diabetic. It has too much carbohydrate content and very little protein to keep you full. Eating these types of food has proven to increase blood sugar levels of diabetics significantly. Stick to a protein-based, low carb breakfast instead.

→ Starchy vegetables such as taro, potatoes, yams and sweet potatoes. Steer clear especially of French fries. Potatoes are already high in carbohydrates; deep-frying them produces toxic chemicals such as aldehydes and advanced glycation end products that are linked to inflammation. Frequent consumption of French fries have been linked to some cancers and heart disease.

→ Beer

→ Milk

→ Sweetened tea, juice, punch and soda: These are high in carbohydrates and loaded with fructose, which has a strong link to insulin resistance and diabetes. Fructose also promotes visceral fat and harmful triglyceride and cholesterol levels. Consuming too much of these beverages could also increase the chances of developing fatty liver. Instead of these beverages, stay hydrated by drinking unsweetened tea, club soda or water.

→ Fruit, especially dried fruit: Dried fruit takes away the water in the fruit and leaves you with a concentrated amount of sugar. Instead of the water in the fruit helping to fill you up, you tend to eat more to compensate when the fruit is dried.

→ Food with trans fats: Trans fats are created when hydrogen is added to unsaturated fatty acids to help extend shelf life of food. While trans fats do not increase your blood sugar, it has been linked to increasing insulin resistance. Baked goods, spreads such as margarine and peanut butter, frozen dinners, creamers and crackers contain trans fats. Check the label and avoid foods that indicate "partially hydrogenated" on the package.

→ Fruit-flavored yogurt: While plain yogurt is healthy for those with diabetes, the fruit-flavored kinds are full of sugar. Stick to whole-milk plain yogurt with no sugar.

→ Flavored coffee: There have been studies that link coffee to some health benefits, including reducing the chances of developing diabetes. Flavored coffee drinks are loaded with sugar, however, and easily raise your blood sugar levels. Keep your coffee order simple to just plain black coffee or an espresso with a little bit of heavy cream or half and half. Do not add sugar.

→ Other forms of sugar such as maple syrup, brown sugar, agave and honey: Even though they are considered natural and unprocessed, they still contain as many carbohydrates as white sugar, sometimes even more. Avoid any kind of sugar and use natural sweeteners that are also low-carb instead, such as stevia, erythritol and xylitol.

→ Packaged snacks: Snacks made from white flour make your blood sugar levels shoot up and have hardly any nutrients in it. It's better to snack on cheese, some low-carb veggies or nuts when you're hungry.

This might seem like a long list, but to sum it up, just avoid food with refined carbohydrates, unhealthy fats, processed grains and liquid or added sugars.

Sample Meal Plans

Low Carb:

	Breakfast	Lunch	Dinner	Snack/ Pre-Workout Food	Total
	Sausage & egg breakfast cup	Cheesy chicken and cauliflower rice	Grilled Beef-Mushroom Burgers	Cauliflower Pizza Muffins	
Calories	502	329	304	164	1.299
Carbohydrates	2 grams	5 grams	7 grams	4 grams	18 grams
Protein	33 grams	31 grams	26 grams	9 grams	99 grams
Fat	39 grams	19 grams	19 grams	12 grams	89 grams

Moderate Carb:

	Breakfast	Lunch	Dinner	Snack/Pre-Workout Food	Total
	Egg & Bacon Pancake Breakfast Wraps	Greens & Grains Pesto Energy Bowl	Moroccan Couscous With Flank Steak	Tex Mex Air Fryer Cauliflower Munchies	
Calories	411	621	371	190	1,593
Carbohydrates	19.1 grams	71 grams	41 grams	11 grams	142.1 grams
Protein	14.3 grams	29 grams	32 grams	3 grams	78.3 grams
Fat	31.1 grams	26 grams	9 grams	16 grams	82.1 grams

High Carb:

	Breakfast	Lunch	Dinner	Snack/Pre-Workout Food	Total
	Red Eye Protein Parfait	Sweet & Spicy Beef Meal	Shrimp Chipotle Bowl	Date & Walnut Energy Snacks	
Calories	521	459	410	188	1,578
Carbohydrates	55 grams	45 grams	56 grams	27 grams	183 grams
Protein	53 grams	40 grams	40 grams	1 gram	134 grams
Fat	10 grams	11 grams	3 grams	10 grams	34 grams

CHAPTER 7: CARB CYCLING-FRIENDLY BREAKFAST RECIPES

Low Carb

Bacon & Eggs

Prep time: 0 minutes

Cook time: 10 minutes

This classic breakfast is easy to make and low in carbohydrates, but very filling with all the eggs and bacon slices. Gauge how hungry you are and adjust the number of eggs as needed. A tomato is added, which adds essential nutrients to your meal, such as vitamin K, C, folate and potassium. But the highlight of this breakfast is the incredible egg. A few years back, many people shunned eating eggs due to the yolk's high cholesterol content. In 2000, the American Heart Association (AHA) deemed eggs healthy for daily consumption. Although even with their revised dietary guidelines, the AHA still advises to keep your cholesterol consumption at 300 mg (a large egg contains about 213 mg) (Zelman, 2007).

Since there is a link between heart disease and high blood cholesterol, people thought eggs were unhealthy to consume. Several years of studies later, it was discovered that saturated fat, which you get from fatty meat and dairy products, triggers production of cholesterol, not cholesterol content.

Eggs contain a lot of protein but are low in calories. They come with other nutrients such as iron, choline, lutein and zeaxanthin. Eggs keep your eyes healthy and enhance brain and memory development. They help in weight loss as they keep you full faster and longer. Egg farmers nowadays have also improved the nutrition in eggs, creating somewhat of a "designer" version. There are now eggs with omega-3 fatty acids, free range eggs or organic eggs.

Servings: 4

Calories: 272

Carbs: 5 grams

Protein: 15 grams

Fat: 22 grams

Ingredients:

→ 6 strips of bacon

→ 8 eggs

→ 1 small tomato (100 grams)

Directions:

1.   On medium high heat, fry the bacon to desired crispiness. Set aside.

2.   Over medium heat, fry the eggs in the bacon grease.

3.   Slice the tomato and fry the slices over medium heat on the bacon grease.

4.   Sprinkle salt and pepper if needed.

Baked Eggs With Tex-Mex Beef Casserole

Prep time: 15 minutes

Cook time: 40 minutes

Easy to make but festive to make your meal feel special. This meal requires tex-mex seasoning. To ensure there is no added sugar, it's best to make this seasoning at home as the store bought ones usually have added sugar.

The recipe calls for beef but you may substitute ground chicken or turkey, but if you want an excellent source of protein, stick with the beef. Aside from protein, beef provides many micronutrients, such a potassium, iron, magnesium, zinc, pantothenate, selenium thiamine, phosphorus, riboflavin, vitamins D, B6, and B12 and niacin. Beef also contains choline and conjugated linoleic acid, which may help decrease the risk of type 2 diabetes and some cancers, and monounsaturated fat, a healthy fat. Lean beef is also very satiating and is nutrient-rich.

Servings: 1

Calories: 655

Carbs: 6 grams

Protein: 41.5 grams

Fat: 50.5 grams

Ingredients:

→ 3 oz ground beef

→ ¼ oz butter

→ ⅓ tbsp Tex-Mex seasoning

→ ¾ oz crushed tomatoes

→ Salt and pepper

→ 2 eggs

→ ¼ oz pickled jalapenos

→ 2 ¾ oz shredded cheese

For topping:

→ Sprinkle of scallions

→ A dollop of crème fraîche or sour cream

→ A dollop of guacamole

→ ½ oz iceberg lettuce or other leafy greens

Directions:

1. Preheat the oven to 400°F.

2. On medium high heat, cook the ground beef in the butter.

3. Add the crushed tomatoes and Tex-Mex seasoning. Stir well until the seasoning and tomatoes are evenly distributed. Let it simmer for 5 minutes. Add salt and pepper if needed.

4. Put the ground beef in a small, greased baking dish. Make two holes in the ground beef and crack the eggs in the holes.

5. Sprinkle the cheese and jalapeños on top.

6. Bake on the top rack until the eggs are cooked, which is around 10 to 15 minutes.

7. Chop the scallions and place in a bowl with the sour cream or crème fraîche.

8. Serve the casserole with a dollop of the scallion and sour cream/crème fraîche mix, some guacamole, and the lettuce/leafy greens on the side.

Frittata With Spinach

Prep time: 10 minutes

Cook time: 35 minutes

Aside from the protein and fat from the bacon/sausage, and eggs, this recipe comes with nutritious, low carb spinach. Anyone familiar with Popeye, the cartoon, knows spinach is chock full of vitamins and minerals. It provides energy to your body, improves your blood quality and increases vitality. Spinach is abundant in iron, which plays the main role in your red blood cells distributing oxygen to your body, in producing energy and in DNA synthesis. Aside from iron, spinach is also full of vitamin B2, vitamin A, magnesium, vitamin C, manganese, folate and vitamin K, which is used to maintain bone health.

Servings: 4

Calories: 661

Carbs: 4 grams

Protein: 27 grams

Fat: 59 grams

Ingredients:

→ 6 strips of bacon or 2 chorizo links, diced

→ 2 tbsp butter

→ 8 oz spinach (fresh)

→ 8 eggs

→ 1 cup heavy whipping cream

→ Salt and pepper

→ 5 oz shredded cheese

Directions:

1. Grease a baking dish (9x9 inches) and preheat your oven to 350°F.

2.   In medium heat, fry the bacon/sausage in the butter to your desired crispiness. Dice the bacon/sausage.

3.   Add the spinach and stir for a few seconds until the leaves wilt. Set aside the bacon/sausage and spinach.

4.   Scramble the eggs and pour in the cream. Sprinkle a little salt and pepper. Mix well. Pour the egg and cream mixture into the baking dish.

5.   Add the bacon/sausage, spinach and shredded cheese. Make sure you spread it evenly in the baking dish.

6.   Place in the middle rack in the oven and bake for 25 to 30 minutes. It is done when the top is golden brown and the middle has set.

Banana Waffles

Prep time: 10 minutes

Cook time: 20 minutes

Did you think with a low carb diet, you'll have to say goodbye to waffles and pancakes for breakfast? Of course not. If you replace regular white flour with another ingredient, such as almond flour, you can enjoy low carb pancakes and waffles, even on your low carb days.

Adding the ground psyllium husk powder to the mix packs your waffles with additional fiber, along with the fiber the banana is already providing. The banana will also provide a lot of potassium, vitamin C, vitamin A, magnesium and vitamin B6 to your breakfast. Vitamin B6 helps by increasing production of white blood cells, reducing inflammation, strengthening your nervous system, aiding in weight loss and guarding against developing type 2 diabetes. Bananas are also high in antioxidants, which can protect you from free radicals. In fact, there is evidence that bananas may prevent kidney cancer, due to those vital antioxidants. They are also better for you as an after-workout snack to replenish your energy and electrolytes than sports drinks because, aside from all the vitamins and minerals mentioned earlier, the antioxidants helps with oxidative stress and helps you improve your performance.

Servings: 8

Calories: 155

Carbs: 4 grams

Protein: 5 grams

Fat: 13 grams

Ingredients:

→ 1 ripe banana, mashed

→ 4 eggs, scrambled
→ ¾ cup almond flour
→ ¾ cup coconut milk
→ 1 tbsp ground psyllium husk powder
→ 1 pinch salt
→ 1 tsp baking powder
→ ½ tsp vanilla extract
→ 1 tsp ground cinnamon
→ Butter or coconut oil

Directions:

1.   Mix all of the ingredients in a bowl, except for the butter/coconut oil.

2.   Grease the waffle iron with the coconut oil or butter.

3.   Pour about ⅓ cup of the waffle mixture into your waffle maker.

Moderate Carb

Heavy Breakfast With Fried Eggs and Yogurt

Prep time: 6 minutes

Cook time: 7 minutes

Adding the yogurt and blueberries to this breakfast increases the amount of carbohydrates in your breakfast, but all the nutrients that come with it make it well worth it. Yogurt provides riboflavin, vitamin B12, phosphorus and calcium. Aside from all these vitamins and minerals, yogurt is also full of probiotics that provide various health benefits from better digestion, to increased immunity and lower cholesterol.

Blueberries, popularly known as a superfood, is a nutrient powerhouse. They are low in calories but one of the most nutrient-dense berries. Blueberries are packed with fiber, manganese, vitamins K and C, and smaller amounts of other nutrients. It also has one of the high levels of antioxidants compared to other produce. Blueberries may help reverse DNA damage, prevent cancer, lessen cholesterol in your blood, lower blood pressure, prevent heart disease, improve memory and brain function. They are also known to improve insulin sensitivity and glucose metabolism, prevent urinary tract infection and lessen the damage to muscles from exercise.

The added walnuts to the yogurt provides a boost of fat and protein with minimal carbohydrates, most of which is fiber. Walnuts contain the omega-3 fat alpha-linolenic acid (ALA), which is healthy for your heart. ALA also improves blood fat composition and reduces inflammation (Arnarson, PhD, 2019). Walnuts also have a high amount of antioxidants compared to other food and helps in improving brain health and preventing cancer and heart disease. Walnuts also provide vitamins and minerals such as vitamin E, copper, manganese, folic acid, vitamin B6 and phosphorus. All these vitamins and minerals improve heart health, strengthen the immune system and support nerve and bone functions. This breakfast is ideal for when you have a moderate amount of activity at the start of your day, giving you the boost of energy to get things done.

Servings: 1

Calories: 1,173

Carbs: 31 grams

Protein: 47 grams

Fat: 95 grams

Ingredients:

→ 2 eggs

→ ½ ounce of butter

→ ½ avocado

→ 1 tomato

→ ½ ounce of baby spinach

→ 1 cup Greek yogurt

→ 2 ounces walnuts

→ 3 ounces of blueberries

→ 1 cup coffee/tea

→ 2 tbsp heavy whipping cream

Directions:

1.   Over medium heat, cook your eggs with the butter. Add salt and pepper to taste.

2.   Plate your eggs with the avocado, tomato, and spinach.

3.   In a separate bowl, pour the yogurt and top with walnuts and blueberries.

4.   Enjoy with a cup of brewed coffee or tea with cream.

Chickpea Flour Pancakes

Prep time: 5 minutes

Cook time: 5 minutes

This is a savory dish that originates from North India. This is a traditional dish normally served for breakfast or brunch. We use chickpea flour for this dish. Chickpea flour is a gluten-free substitute for wheat flour, is less energy dense, meaning it has fewer calories and is higher in fiber and protein. It also has a lower GI level compared to wheat flour. Chickpeas are rich in nutrients such as manganese, thiamine, copper, folate, magnesium, iron and phosphorus. To illustrate how nutritious chickpeas are, one cup of chickpeas provides 101 percent of the recommended daily allowance (RDA) of folate, 74 percent of the RDA of manganese, and 42 percent of the RDA of copper (Shoemaker, MS, RDN, LD, 2019).

Chickpeas are also high in antioxidants that may help reduce damage from free radicals. Using chickpea flour in processed food reduces the amount of acrylamide, which may cause cancer and problems with muscle and nerve function and reproduction, and hormone and enzyme activity.

Servings: 4

Calories: 253

Carbs: 33.8 grams

Protein: 10.1 grams

Fat: 10.1 grams

Ingredients:

→ 1 tbsp olive oil (you may also use ghee)

→ ½ tsp pepper

→ 1 cup chickpea flour (also known as garbanzo or besan flour)
→ ½ tsp salt
→ 1 tsp turmeric
→ 1 cup water
→ 3 spring onions, finely diced
Directions:
1.   Heat the olive oil in a non-stick frying pan. Make sure the pan is coated well with oil before you start cooking.
2.   Combine the pepper, flour, salt, turmeric, and water in a blender or food processor. Make sure the batter is very runny. Add the spring onions.
3.   On medium heat, pour about ½ cup of the mixture onto the hot pan and let it cook for 3 minutes.
4.   Flip the pancake over and cook for another 3 minutes. Add more oil to the pan if needed.

Banana Egg Pancakes

Prep time: 3 minutes

Cook time: 7 minutes

This is a good dish to eat before going for your cardio workout. This recipe just requires three ingredients and 10 minutes of your time. You'll get all the nutrients and health benefits from the eggs and bananas in this tasty dish.

Servings: 1

Calories: 231

Carbs: 28 grams

Protein: 12 grams

Fat: 9 grams

Ingredients:

→ 1 ripe banana, mashed

→ 2 eggs, scrambled

→ Oil or butter

Directions:

1. Combine the eggs and banana.

2. Over low heat, heat up the oil/butter in a frying pan and fry the egg/banana mixture, cooking for about a minute or two per side.

High Carb

Dutch Apple Pancake

Prep time: 5 minutes

Cook time: 20 minutes

Do you need a big energy boost for your morning? This pancake packs 78.5 grams of carbohydrates to fuel your body. This recipe uses your choice of apple though we recommend Granny Smith or Golden Delicious. Apples provide your body with vitamin C, phytochemicals and fiber, especially when you eat it with the skin on. By discarding the skin, you deprive yourself with most of the flavonoids and fiber that come with this type of fruit. Apples also have a low GI. Studies have shown that including apples in your diet helps improve your cardiovascular health, reduce the risk of type 2 diabetes and cancer, and help you control your weight (*Apples*, 2018).

Servings: 2

Calories: 477

Carbs: 78.5 grams

Protein: 14 grams

Fat: 12.7 grams

Ingredients:

→ 1 apple

→ 1 tbsp butter

→ 1 tbsp maple syrup + 1 tbsp

→ ¾ cups wheat flour

→ 2 eggs

→ 1 tsp lemon zest

→ 1 tbsp lemon juice

→ ¼ tsp salt

→ 1 tsp cinnamon

→ ½ cup milk

Directions:

1. Preheat the oven to 340°F.

2. Slice the apple thinly. If you can, leave the skin on to add to your fiber intake.

3. Over a medium heat, caramelize the butter, half of the maple syrup and the apple slices in a non-stick, oven-proof pan for 5 minutes.

4. Using a hand blender, add the flour, eggs, lemon zest and lemon juice, the rest of the maple syrup, salt, cinnamon and milk to make the batter. Mix well and make sure the batter is lump-free.

5. Pour the batter into the pan and cook for 2 minutes, then place the pan in the oven for 12 minutes.

Ironman Oatmeal

Prep time: 5 minutes

Cook time: 5 minutes

As the name suggests, this breakfast food aims to help you conquer a very tough, very physical day that requires you to have a lot of energy. This dish features oatmeal - made up of oats, one of the healthiest grains. Oats are nutrient-dense, packed with antioxidants, vitamins, fiber and minerals. As a regular part of your diet, they can reduce the risk of heart disease, lower blood pressure and cholesterol levels, help with lowering your blood sugar, increase the growth of good bacteria in your gut and aid in weight loss.

A ½ cup of oats can provide you with 191 percent of the recommended daily allowance (RDA) of manganese, four percent of the RDI of phosphorus, and 34 percent of the RDI of magnesium, along with numerous other vitamins and minerals (Palsdottir, MS, 2016).

Servings: 1

Calories: 452

Carbs: 50 grams

Protein: 13 grams

Fat: 24 grams

Ingredients:

→ 2 tbsp chopped almonds

→ 1 tbsp dried apricots sliced into bite-size pieces

→ ½ cup rolled oats

→ 1 tbsp coconut flakes

→ 1 tbsp sunflower seeds

→ ½ tsp cinnamon

→ 1 cup almond milk

Directions:

1.   Combine all the ingredients together.

2.   Mix well then serve.

Carrot Cake Protein Oatmeal

Prep time: 5 minutes

Cook time: 5 minutes

This high-carb breakfast option turns into high-protein with the addition of whey protein powder. This recipe calls for carrots. Carrots are root vegetables full of antioxidants, beta carotene, potassium, fiber, and vitamin K1. Raw carrots rank low on the GI. Carrots can improve eye health, help you lose weight, lower your cholesterol and your risk of developing certain cancers. (Bjarnadottir, MS, RDN (Ice), 2019).

Servings: 1

Calories: 439

Carbs: 50 grams

Protein: 34 grams

Fat: 15 grams

Ingredients:

→ 1 scoop vanilla whey protein powder

→ 3 oz unsweetened almond milk

→ ½ cup cooked dry oats

→ 3 tbsp shredded carrots

→ Dash of allspice

→ Dash of cinnamon

→ Dash of nutmeg

→ 1 tbsp maple syrup/honey/stevia/agave

Directions:

1.   Mix the protein powder with the almond milk until well blended. Combine with the cooked oatmeal.

2.   Add the carrots, spices, and maple syrup to the oatmeal mix and blend well.

CHAPTER 8: CARB CYCLING-FRIENDLY LUNCH/DINNER RECIPES

Low Carb

Cheesy Chicken and Rice

Prep time: 20 minutes

Cook time: 20 minutes

The use of cauliflower rice instead of white or brown rice makes this dish a low carb version that doesn't sacrifice taste. Cauliflower rice only has 5 grams per cup versus 46 grams in 1 cup of white or brown rice. It is also lower in calories compared to brown rice - one cup of cauliflower rice has only 25 calories, compared to one cup of brown rice which has 218 calories (Lipton, 2016). The instructions below will show you how easy it is to make cauliflower rice. Cauliflower gives off a pungent smell when cooked however, so don't cook it for too long if you don't like the smell.

Cauliflower is rich in fiber, folate and vitamins K and C. It is also full of antioxidants and phytochemicals. Cauliflower is so good for you. It ranks in the top 25 of the Aggregate Nutrient Density Index, a list compiled by the Centers for Disease Control and Prevention which ranks food based on how nutritious it is per calorie (Szalay, 2018). Including cauliflower in your diet can help reduce the risks of some cancers and cardiovascular disease, and improve your digestive health.

Servings: 4

Calories: 329

Carbs: 5 grams

Protein: 31 grams

Fat: 19 grams

Ingredients:
- → ½ head cauliflower cut to even-sized pieces
- → 1 tbsp olive oil + 1 tbsp + 1 tbsp
- → salt and pepper
- → 4 cups broccoli cut to bite-sized pieces
- → 1 lb boneless, skinless chicken breasts cut to bite-sized pieces
- → ¼ tsp pepper
- → 1 tsp onion powder
- → ¼ tsp salt
- → 1 tsp garlic powder
- → 1 cup shredded cheese

Directions:

1. Either in a food processor or using a box grater, break down your cauliflower to make rice.

2. Over low heat, heat 1 tbsp olive oil and when hot, cook your cauliflower rice until slightly soft (about 5 minutes). Season with salt and pepper. Set aside.

3. Heat 1 tbsp of olive oil in your pan and once hot, sauté the broccoli for 5-7 minutes to your desired softness. Place on top of the cauliflower rice and set aside.

4. Heat the remaining 1 tbsp of olive oil in your pan and once hot, sauté the chicken with the pepper, onion powder, salt, and garlic powder until cooked all the way through (about 7 to 10 minutes). Place on top of the cauliflower rice and broccoli. Top with the shredded cheese.

Santa Fe Chicken

Prep time: 15 minutes

Cook time: 15 minutes

This dish has a Mexican influence with the use of taco seasoning and cilantro leaves. To make sure your taco seasoning doesn't have any added sugar to it, it's best to make it yourself, or check the label if store-bought.

Cilantro leaves provide additional fiber content to the dish along with a small boost of other vitamins and minerals such as manganese, vitamins K, A, C, B6, and E, copper, riboflavin, potassium, niacin, phosphorus, magnesium, folate, iron, calcium and pantothenic acid.

Servings: 4

Calories: 303

Carbs: 11 grams

Protein: 28 grams

Fat: 16 grams

Ingredients:

→ 1 tbsp olive oil + 1 tbsp + 1 tbsp

→ 4 cups cauliflower cut to even-sized pieces

→ zest of 1 lime

→ ¼ tsp garlic powder

→ ¼ tsp salt

→ ¼ cup cilantro leaves

→ ½ sliced red onion

→ 2 sliced bell peppers

→ 14 oz chicken breasts, horizontally sliced

→ 2 tbsp taco seasoning

→ ¼ cup shredded cheese

→ 2 avocados (optional)

Directions:

1.   Either in a food processor or using a box grater, break down your cauliflower to make rice.

2.   Over low heat, heat 1 tbsp of olive oil in a pan and once hot, add the cauliflower, lime zest, garlic powder and salt. Cook to your desired softness (around 5 minutes). Stir in the cilantro, place on a plate and set aside.

3.   Heat up 1 tbsp of olive oil in the pan and once hot, sauté the onion and bell peppers for 5 minutes. Place on top of the cauliflower rice.

4.   Brush the chicken breasts with 1 tbsp olive oil and season with taco seasoning.

5.   Cook the chicken all the way through in the pan.

6.   Place the cooked chicken on top of the cauliflower rice and top with the shredded cheese. You may add fresh, sliced avocados on the side.

Indian Chicken Skillet

Prep time: 15 minutes

Cook time: 10 minutes

Cooked with traditional Indian spices, this chicken skillet dish is packed with flavor as much as it is packed with nutrients. This dish makes use of various spices, all of which bring its own health benefits. Take cumin, for example. Cumin can help relieve symptoms of a common cold, help control your blood pressure, reduce digestive problems, and reduce the risk of getting anemia. Garam masala, a mix of different spices that may include bay leaves, cloves, cardamom, cinnamon, peppercorn, nutmeg, and cumin, helps with digestion, fights bloating, may help you lose weight by increasing your metabolism, and help reduce inflammation.

Servings: 4

Calories: 207

Carbs: 8 grams

Protein: 24 grams

Fat: 8 grams

Ingredients:

→ 1 tbsp olive oil

→ 1 lb boneless, skinless chicken thighs

→ salt and pepper

→ ¼ cup of water

→ ½ tsp salt

→ 1 tsp cumin

→ ⅓ tsp garam masala

→ 1 tsp curry powder

→ ½ tsp ground coriander

→ ½ tsp onion powder

→ ½ tsp garlic powder

→ ¼ cup tomato sauce

→ 4 cups cauliflower cut to even-sized pieces

→ 1 ½ cups fresh green beans

Directions:

1.   Heat the olive oil in a frying pan. Once hot, cook the chicken until the inside is no longer pink (about 5 minutes each side) and season with salt and pepper to taste. Set aside on a plate.

2.   Pour the water and the ½ tsp salt, cumin, garam masala, curry powder, coriander, onion powder and garlic powder in the pan and stir until the spices are blended well. With constant stirring, let the mixture simmer for 2 minutes.

3.   Add the tomato sauce, making sure the spices are well blended.

4.   Either in a food processor or using a box grater, break down your cauliflower to make rice.

5.   Mix in the cauliflower rice to the pan and stir until the tomato sauce, spices, and cauliflower rice are well blended.

6.   Add the green beans to the pot and cook to desired tenderness.

Sesame Ginger Beef With Noodles

Prep time: 10 minutes

Cook time: 10 minutes

This Asian-inspired dish uses spiralized zucchini instead of regular wheat pasta. Zucchinis are lower in calories compared to brussel sprouts or broccoli. They contain nutrients such as iron, potassium, vitamin A and C and folate. It is low carb but high in water content, filling you up faster as well as keeping your body hydrated.

Servings: 4

Calories: 381

Carbs: 5 grams

Protein: 21 grams

Fat: 30 grams

Ingredients:

→ 1 tbsp monk fruit sweetener or ⅛ tbsp liquid Stevia

→ 2 tbsp apple cider vinegar

→ ¼ cup low sodium soy sauce

→ 1 lb ground beef

→ 3 cloves minced garlic

→ 1 tbsp fresh, finely-grated ginger

→ 2 tbsp toasted sesame oil

→ 2 medium spiralized zucchinis

Directions:

1.   Mix the monk fruit sweetener/stevia, apple cider vinegar and soy sauce in a bowl and set aside.

2.   Over medium heat, cook the beef on a heated non-stick pan until no longer pink. Drain oil if needed.

3.   Add the garlic, ginger and sesame oil to the beef and let it cook for 1 minute, blending all the ingredients well.

4.   Add the sauce to the pan and let it cook for 1 minute, making sure to coat the beef well.

5.   Steam or boil the zucchini for one minute.

6.   Top the spiralized zucchinis with the cooked beef and serve.

Moderate Carb

Harira

Prep time: 20 minutes

Cook time: 2 hours 25 minutes

This recipe takes a while to cook to make sure the lamb is tender, but if you have a pressure cooker, feel free to use it to cut down on the cooking time. You may also substitute lamb for beef or chicken if you don't like the gamey flavor of lamb. But do consider making this soup with lamb as it provides high amounts of protein, the nine essential amino acids your body needs, and other essential vitamins and minerals, such as iron, vitamin B12, phosphorus, selenium, niacin, and zinc. Lamb, like any other kind of red meat, is important in muscle repair, healing, muscle function and improved physical performance. Meat is also the best source of iron, which prevents anemia.

While lamb has a slightly higher level of saturated fat compared to pork and beef, it has the highest amount of conjugated linoleic acid (CLA), a type of ruminant trans fat that helps in weight loss.

Servings: 6

Calories: 515

Carbs: 31 grams

Protein: 39 grams

Fat: 24 grams

Ingredients:

→ 700g diced lamb shoulder

→ Salt and pepper

→ 2 tbsp olive oil

→ 2 chopped garlic cloves

→ 1 chopped onion

→ 1/2 tsp ground cloves

→ 2 tsp sweet paprika

→ 1 ½ tsp ground cumin

→ 1 bay leaf

→ 2 tbsp tomato paste

→ ½ bunch finely chopped coriander

→ 800 grams canned chopped tomatoes

→ 1 liter beef stock

→ 800 grams canned brown lentils, rinsed and drained

→ 800 grams canned chickpeas, rinsed and drained

Seasoning for the lamb (optional):

- ⅛ tsp dry ginger powder
- ⅛ tsp turkish oregano
- ⅛ tsp dried spearmint leaves
- ⅛ tsp dried rosemary
- ⅛ tsp garlic powder
- ⅛ tsp cumin
- ⅛ tsp onion powder
- ⅛ tsp celery seed
- ⅛ tsp black pepper
- ⅛ tsp paprika

Directions:

1. Season the lamb. You may use just salt and pepper, but to really bring out the flavor of the lamb and the meat's richness, we recommend you use a mix of dry ginger powder, turkish oregano, dried spearmint

leaves, dried rosemary, garlic powder, cumin, onion powder, celery seed, black pepper, paprika, salt and pepper.

2.   Over medium-high heat, heat the olive oil in a saucepan. Once hot enough, place the seasoned lamb in the pan and cook for 4 to 5 minutes on both sides until the meat turns brown. Set the lamb aside.

3.   Sauté the onion and garlic until fragrant and soft. Place the lamb back in the pan and add the ground cloves, paprika, ground cumin, bay leaf and tomato paste. Stir and cook for 1 minute.

4.   Add the coriander, canned tomatoes and beef stock, simmer, cover and turn down the heat to low. Let the meat cook for at least 1 hour to make it tender.

5.   Add the canned lentils and chickpeas, cover and continue cooking for 30 minutes.

6.   Uncover and cook for another 30 minutes until the sauce has thickened.

7.   You may serve with pita bread and yogurt on the side.

Carrot, Ginger and Lentil Soup

Prep time: 10 minutes

Cook time: 2 hours

A delicious vegan soup that has carrots, ginger, and French lentils. If you've never tried French lentils before, do so now with this dish. French lentils are a type of green lentils, but with a darker color and a size that is about one-third the diameter of the average green lentil. French lentils are good to use in soups and salads because they hold their shape very well and don't turn into mush after cooking. Flavorwise, compared to the standard green lentil, French lentils have an earthy, peppery nutty flavor.

Servings: 4

Calories: 261

Carbs: 32.9 grams

Protein: 10.6 grams

Fat: 10.7 grams

Ingredients:

→ Salt and pepper

→ 6 large carrots, chopped to large pieces

→ ½ tsp fennel seeds

→ 2 tbsp olive oil + 1 tbsp

→ 3 thinly-sliced garlic cloves

→ 1 chopped onion

→ 2 chopped celery stalks

→ ¼ tbsp grated ginger

→ Leaves from 3 sprigs of thyme

→ 6 cups vegetable stock

→ 1 cup French lentils

→ 2 ½ cups of cold water

Directions:

1. Preheat the oven to 350°F.

2. In a bowl, season and toss carrots, and fennel seeds with 2 tbsp of olive oil.

3. Place in a baking tray lined with baking paper and roast in the oven until desired tenderness (about 30 minutes).

4. Over medium heat, pour 1 tbsp olive oil in a saucepan. Once hot, sauté the garlic and onion until soft and fragrant (about 3 to 4 minutes). Add the celery and let it cook until soft (about 3 to 4 minutes). Add the roasted carrots, grated ginger, thyme, and vegetable stock. Cook for 25 to 30 minutes, occasionally stirring .

5. While the carrots and ginger are cooking, in a separate saucepan, boil lentils in 2 ½ cups of water. Turn down the heat to low and cook until the lentils have absorbed the water and have become tender (about 30 minutes).

6. Pour the cooked carrots and ginger mix into a blender and puree until smooth in consistency.

7. Pour the pureed carrots in the saucepan where the lentils are cooking and stir. Turn up to medium heat and cook for an additional 2 minutes, stirring occasionally, then remove from heat.

8. Optional: Serve the soup with some type of crusty bread.

Pea and Ham Soup With Salami Pesto Puff Pastry

Prep time: 15 minutes

Cook time: 15 minutes

The freshly baked salami pesto puff pastry pairs really well with the warm, comforting bowl of pea and ham soup. The peas in this recipe adds additional starch to the dish, providing you with added energy for a moderate-intensity workout. Aside from supplying you with energy, peas also have a good protein content, but are low in calories. They also have a lot of vitamin K, important for blood clotting and keeping your bones healthy. Peas also have fiber, manganese, vitamins A and C, thiamin, folate, iron and has a low GI level. Consuming peas regularly will help you control your blood sugar and help you lose weight as it is a very filling but low-calorie food. Since it also has fiber, peas can help improve your digestive health and lower your blood pressure due to their mineral content and antioxidants.

Servings: 6

Calories: 512

Carbs: 32 grams

Protein: 15 grams

Fat: 35 grams

Ingredients:

→ 50 grams unsalted butter

→ 1 finely chopped onion

→ 225 grams chopped potatoes

→ 900 ml chicken stock

→ 350 grams frozen peas

→ 100 grams thinly-sliced leg ham

→ 1 tbsp chopped mint

→ 1 tbsp chopped Italian parsley

→ 150 ml thick cream
→ 2 sheets puff pastry
→ 1 tbsp basil pesto
→ 1 tbsp sun-dried tomato pesto
→ 100 grams salami

Directions:

1. Preheat the oven to 350°F.
2. Over low heat, melt the butter in a saucepan and add the onion. Cook the onion until transparent.
3. Add the potatoes and sauté for 1 to 2 minutes.
4. Add the chicken stock and cook the potatoes until soft (about 10 minutes).
5. Add and boil the peas (about 3 minutes).
6. Pour the contents of the saucepan into a blender and puree until consistency is smooth. Place back in the saucepan.
7. Add the ham and sprinkle with salt and pepper.
8. Add the mint, Italian parsley and cream, then stir until well blended and heated through.
9. Place the puff pastry on top of a baking pan lined with baking paper. Poke small holes in the puff pastry with a fork and bake in the oven for 5 minutes.
10. Spread the basil pesto on top of one sheet of puff pastry and the tomato pesto on top of the other sheet of puff pastry.
11. Lay the salami on top of each sheet of puff pastry and bake until the puff pastry is golden in color (about 10 minutes).
12. Slice each puff pastry sheet in half then cut further into 1-inch strips. Serve the salami pesto puff pastry with the pea and ham soup.

High Carb

Lentil and Brown Rice Salad

Prep time: 15 minutes

Cook time: 0 minutes

This energy-dense salad will give you the boost of energy you need to conquer your high-intensity workout. This salad includes a hefty serving of lentils - a low fat, low calorie, complex carb. Lentils also have a low GI value, making them an ideal food for those with diabetes. Lentils are high in protein and high in fiber, providing 32 percent of the recommended daily allowance for fiber. Out of all plant-based foods, lentils have the most folate content, which supports nerve functions and red blood cell formation. It also prevents anemia due to its high iron content and reduces the risk of dementia, some cancers, and heart disease. Because it is a good source of manganese, lentils can help increase insulin sensitivity.

Servings: 6

Calories: 430

Carbs: 45 grams

Protein: 12 grams

Fat: 20 grams

Ingredients:

→ 1 tbsp Dijon mustard

→ ⅓ cup olive oil

→ 2 tbsp red wine vinegar

→ Salt and pepper

→ 1 small finely diced red onion

→ 400 g canned brown lentils, drained and rinsed

→ 2 cups cooked long grain brown rice

→ 400 g canned borlotti beans, drained and rinsed

→ 2 tbsp chopped flat-leaf parsley

→ 2 hearts of radicchio, shredded

→ ¼ cup chopped fresh tarragon

→ 2 finely chopped tomatoes

Directions:

1.   In a bowl, blend the mustard, oil and vinegar. Season with salt and pepper to taste.

2.   In a separate bowl, combine onion, lentils, rice, beans, parsley, shredded radicchio, tarragon and tomatoes.

3.   Toss the vegetables with the dressing.

Char Siu Beef With Broccolini

Prep time: 15 minutes

Cook time: 10 minutes

This dish includes broccolini - a cross-breed of broccoli and Chinese kale. This vegetable is full of beta-carotene, which promotes healthy skin, and antioxidants that protect your skin from free radicals and reduce the risk of some cancers. Broccolini also has vitamin C, which boosts your immune system and reduces inflammation, and potassium, which improves heart health. This vegetable is also high in fiber and feeds the good bacteria in your gut. Broccolini also helps detoxify your liver and balance your hormones (*4 Health Benefits Of Broccolini*, 2019).

Servings: 4

Calories: 500

Carbs: 42 grams

Protein: 28 grams

Fat: 22 grams

Ingredients:

→ 100g thin rice noodles

→ 1 tbsp sunflower oil

→ 2 chopped garlic cloves

→ 2 cm piece ginger, grated

→ 400g ground beef

→ ¼ cup char siu sauce/Chinese barbecue sauce

→ ¼ cup Chinese rice wine

→ 2 bunches broccolini, trimmed, blanched, refreshed

Directions:
1. Cook the rice noodles per package instructions. Drain and set aside.
2. Over high heat, heat the sunflower oil in a wok and once hot, sauté the chopped garlic and grated ginger for a minute.
3. Add the ground beef and brown in the wok.
4. Add the char siu sauce and rice wine. Let it simmer for 1 minute.
5. Add the broccolini and cook until desired tenderness.
6. Top the cooked rice noodles with the beef and broccolini.

Sake Chicken With Buckwheat Noodles

Prep time: 10 minutes

Cook time: 40 minutes

This comforting soup is high in carbs and protein to fill you up quickly. The soup contains both shiitake and enoki mushrooms. Shiitake mushrooms are pretty common, especially in East Asian dishes. Their nutrients help keep your heart healthy, boost your immune system and reduce the risk of getting some cancers. Shiitake mushrooms are high in fiber, and contain a significant amount of B vitamins, yet low in calories. In one serving of dried shiitake (4 pieces or 15 grams), you can get 39 percent of the daily value of copper and 33 percent of the daily value of vitamin B5, along with other vitamins and minerals. Shiitake mushrooms also contain the same amino acids found in meat.

Enoki mushrooms are used frequently in Japanese cuisine, particularly in soups. They contain nutrients such as copper, vitamins B1, B2, B3, and B5, calcium, phosphorus, thiamin, selenium, iron, fiber and amino acids. Enoki mushrooms are also low in cholesterol. Consumption of enoki mushrooms boosts your immune system and metabolism, which may help you lose weight. It also improves your digestive function and balances your blood sugar.

Servings: 4

Calories: 460

Carbs: 57.8 grams

Protein: 41.9 grams

Fat: 4.2 grams

Ingredients:

→ 20g dried shiitake mushrooms

→ ½ cup sake
→ ¼ cup light soy sauce
→ 1 ½ tsp caster sugar
→ 2 cups chicken stock
→ 2 chicken breast fillets (around 180 grams per piece)
→ 1 bunch bok choy
→ 270g soba noodles
→ 150g enoki mushrooms
→ 1 long red chili, thinly sliced

Directions:

1.   Rehydrate the shiitake mushrooms by placing them in a bowl and covering with two cups of hot water. Cover the bowl with a lid or plastic wrap to keep the heat from escaping. Let it sit for about 20 minutes. Take out the mushrooms, but save the liquid.

2.   Combine the mushroom liquid, sake, chicken stock, soy sauce and sugar in a pan let it simmer and occasionally stir.

3.   Add the chicken, let it simmer for 10 minutes.

4.   Turn the chicken pieces over, add the bok choy and cook it through (for about 5 to 7 more minutes).

5.   Once cooked, take out the bok choy and chicken and set aside.

6.   Let the broth simmer again, then add the noodles, shiitake, and enoki mushrooms. Cook until the noodles are to your desired tenderness.

What were your favorite recipes from this book? Write a review on Amazon and tell us about it.

CHAPTER 9: CARB CYCLING-FRIENDLY SNACKS
Low Carb

Salt and Vinegar Zucchini Chips

Prep time: 15 minutes

Cook time: 3 to 14 hours depending on the method you use

Craving potato chips? Keep it healthy and low carb by using zucchini instead of potato. While it takes some time to dry out the zucchini before you can enjoy the chips, we suggest making a big batch and storing them in an airtight container to enjoy over the next few weeks.

Servings: 8

Calories: 40

Carbs: 2.9 grams

Protein: 0.7 grams

Fat: 3.6 grams

Ingredients:

→ 4 cups zucchini, thinly sliced

→ 2 tbsp white balsamic vinegar

→ 2 tbsp extra virgin olive oil

→ 2 tsp coarse sea salt

Directions:

1.   Slice the zucchini as thinly as you possibly can. It would be best to use a mandoline slicer if you have one available. Place the zucchini slices in a large bowl.

2.   Combine the vinegar and olive oil in a large bowl.

3.   Toss the zucchini slices and olive oil/vinegar mixture together.

4.   Sprinkle the sea salt on the zucchini slices.

5.   You may make the zucchini chips in a dehydrator or baked in the oven. If you opt you use a dehydrator, the drying time will depend on how thin the zucchini has been sliced. So at 135°F, it may take anywhere from 8 to 14 hours to dry out the zucchini chips.

6.   You may also use your oven. Place baking paper on a baking tray and place the zucchini slices on top. Keep the oven temperature low (around 200°F) and leave the zucchini chips in for 2 to 3 hours, rotating the chips about 1 to 1 ½ hours into cooking. You will need an oven thermometer to monitor the temperature in the oven. It would also be good to have an oven fan to keep the air circulating on the chip. If no oven fan is available, open the oven door from time to time while the chips are drying out to help the air circulate.

Easy Granola

Prep time: 5 minutes

Cook time: 25 minutes

This is a simple recipe to make and since you're making it at home you can customize it to your liking. For instance, you may add dried fruit such as blueberries for added antioxidants, sunflower seeds for additional crunch or cinnamon for that extra kick. You may also opt to use agave or honey instead of maple syrup. If you want a higher carb granola, add more dried fruit. If you want more protein, you can add more seeds and nuts. And if you want more fiber, increase the whole grains in the mix.

Granola is high in protein and fiber, which can fill you up quickly and for a longer period of time, which may contribute to weight loss. The fiber in the granola may also reduce your blood pressure and cholesterol levels. Other health benefits include improving your blood sugar level, improving your digestive health and reducing inflammation due to the antioxidants found in the ingredients used for granola.

Servings: 20

Calories: 205

Carbs: 9.2 grams

Protein: 4.2 grams

Fat: 18 grams

Ingredients:

→ ¼ tsp sea salt

→ ½ cup coconut flakes (unsweetened)

→ 2 tbsp muscovado, cane or coconut sugar

→ 1 cup raw walnuts

→ 1 ¼ cup raw pecans

→ 2 cups raw almonds (slivered)

→ 1 tbsp flaxseed meal

→ 3 tbsp chia seeds

→ 3 tbsp olive oil or coconut oil

→ ⅓ cup maple syrup

Directions:

1.   Preheat your oven to 325°F.

2.   Combine the salt, coconut, sugar, walnuts, pecans, almonds, flax seeds and chia seeds in a bowl. Mix well.

3.   Heat the maple syrup and olive oil in a saucepan and pour over the nuts mixture in the bowl. Mix well making sure the dry ingredients get coated by the syrup.

4.   Evenly distribute the mixture on a baking sheet and bake in the oven for 20 minutes, then increase the heat to 340°F and bake until golden brown (another 5 to 8 minutes). If using coconut oil instead of olive oil, keep an eye while the granola is baking as the coconut oil browns and burns easily.

5.   Once done, let the granola cool before storing in an airtight container. The granola should last in this type of storage for a few weeks.

Strawberry Cream Cheese Cups

Prep time: 15 minutes

Cook time: 2 hours

This refreshing frozen snack is really easy to make. The recipe calls for fresh strawberries. These bright red, juicy, and sweet fruits are full of Vitamin C, manganese, B9, potassium and antioxidants. The nutrients in strawberries help keep your blood sugar under control, decrease the risks of developing some cancers and keep your heart healthy. Strawberries have a low GI score and low carb content, wherein a quarter of the carbs are made up of fiber.

Servings: 12

Calories: 105

Carbs: 2 grams

Protein: 1 gram

Fat: 10 grams

Ingredients:

→ 1 cup diced strawberries

→ ¾ cup softened cream cheese

→ ¼ cup coconut oil

→ 1 tsp vanilla extract

Directions:

1.   Puree the strawberries in a blender.

2.   Add the cream cheese, coconut oil and vanilla extract. Puree until mixture is smooth in texture.

3.   Grease a 12-cup muffin tin with the coconut oil and pour the strawberry/cream cheese puree in the muffin tins.

4.   Place in the freezer until solid. This should be ready to eat in about 2 hours.

5.   Keep them stored in the freezer.

Parmesan Cheese Chips

Prep time: 10 minutes

Cook time: 7 minutes

These parmesan cheese chips are not just low carb - they are NO CARB! They are easy and quick to make when you need something to munch on during the day between meals. You can substitute any hard cheese like aged cheddar or asiago instead of parmesan. When selecting cheese, the rule of thumb is, the harder a cheese is, the more protein it has and lower in fat. We chose parmesan, however, because it has no carbs and is lactose-free. Aside from fat and protein, parmesan has copper, calcium, zinc, phosphorus and vitamins A, B6, and B12. Because of its high calcium content, parmesan supports your healthy bones.

Servings: 12

Calories: 31

Carbs: 0 grams

Protein: 2 grams

Fat: 2 grams

Ingredients:

→ 1 cup parmesan cheese (shredded)

→ 1 tsp dried basil

Directions:

1.   Preheat your oven to 350°F.

2.   Place piles of shredded parmesan cheese (about 1 tbsp) on a baking tray lined with baking paper, about two inches apart. Flatten each pile with a spoon.

3.   Season with basil.

4.   Place in the oven and bake until golden brown and edges get crispy (about 5 to 7 minutes).

Moderate Carb
Soft Pretzels

Prep time: 45 minutes

Cook time: 25 minutes

These pretzels are gluten-free and low carb. These are also high in fiber because of the psyllium husk powder in the ingredients. Psyllium comes from the husk of the seeds of the Plantago ovata. It improves your digestive health and is a prebiotic, so it strengthens your immune system. Regular intake of psyllium can also lower cholesterol levels, lower the risk of heart disease and help balance your blood sugar levels. Psyllium is fiber and absorbs the water in your body, making you feel full, which may lead to consuming fewer calories.

Servings: 8

Calories: 200

Carbs: 19 grams

Protein: 15 grams

Fat: 7 grams

Ingredients:

→ 1 tbsp active dry yeast

→ 3 tbsp Psyllium powder

→ 1 tbsp natural butter flavor

→ 1 cup unsweetened vanilla almond milk

→ 5 large egg whites

→ ½ cup unsweetened apple sauce

→ ¼ tsp salt

→ 1 ½ cups organic soy flour

→ ½ tsp baking soda

→ 2 tsp double-acting baking powder

→ 1 ¼ cups coconut flour

→ 1 egg yolk

→ 1 tsp water

→ 1 tsp flaked sea salt

Directions:

1. Preheat your oven to 350°F.

2. Combine the yeast and psyllium powder in one bowl.

3. Using a mixer on medium speed, combine the butter flavor, almond milk, egg whites and applesauce. Add the yeast/psyllium powder mixture and mix until it looks like thick gravy.

4. Combine salt, soy flour, baking soda, baking powder, and coconut flour in a separate bowl and blend well. Add this to the mixture in the other bowl using a mixer on low speed until the dough is sticky and very thick and dense.

5. Form the dough into a ball and place in a bowl. Cover the bowl with plastic wrap and leave in a warm area for 1 hour to keep the yeast active.

6. Combine the egg yolk with water and mix well.

7. Divide the dough into 8 equal parts and roll each part into long logs, then shape into pretzels. Place each pretzel on a baking tray lined with baking paper.

8. Brush the pretzels with the egg yolk/water mixture then sprinkle with the flaked sea salt.

9. Place the tray in the oven and let the pretzels bake until golden brown (about 23 to 25 minutes). Serve the pretzels warm.

Peanut Butter Coconut Cookies

Prep time: 10 minutes

Cook time: 20 minutes

These easy-to-make cookies are no bake. Aside from peanut butter, this recipe calls for coconut, the fruit of the coconut palm, which grows in tropical countries. The coconut has many uses – the edible kernel, or meat, has a firm consistency and slightly sweet taste. Coconut cream and coconut milk can be extracted from the kernel by pressing on it. Coconut oil can also be extracted from the kernel. The meat can be shaved or grated, then dried and ground into flour.

For this recipe, we will use coconut oil and flakes. Coconut is mostly fat and has a high manganese content, which is good for your metabolism and healthy bones. It also contains a lot of copper and iron, which is good for red blood cell production. Because coconut is high in fiber, it can help decrease insulin resistance and help control blood sugar, in part due to the amino acid, arginine, which pancreatic cells use to function. Coconut also has antioxidants that help protect from cell damage. Beware however, since coconut is high in fat and calories, which may cause weight gain.

Servings: 8

Calories: 332

Carbs: 19 grams

Protein: 8 grams

Fat: 26 grams

Ingredients:

→ 2 tbsp coconut oil

→ ⅔ cup natural peanut butter

→ 1 tsp vanilla extract

→ 1 cup unsweetened shredded coconut flakes

Directions:

1. Microwave the coconut oil and peanut butter in a bowl for 30 seconds. Stir, then add the vanilla extract. Stir some more until the mixture is well blended.

2. Add the coconut flakes and mix well.

3. On a baking pan lined with baking paper, drop a glob of the mixture that is around 1 ½ inches wide.

4. Freeze for about 15 to 20 minutes until the cookies are solid.

5. Store in an airtight container in the refrigerator.

Plantains With Cinnamon

Prep time: 5 minutes

Cook time: 10 minutes

This is a quick and easy snack to prepare and eat before or after working out. For additional flavor, you may add sugar-free maple syrup, or even real maple syrup or honey, keeping in mind not to go overboard since the plantains already contain natural sugar.

Plantains look like bananas but are starchier and less sweet-tasting. They have to be cooked before eaten. Plantains are made up mostly of carbohydrates, but complex carbs. They contain antioxidants, potassium, fiber, magnesium and vitamins A, B6, and C (Cafasso & Marengo, LDN, RD, 2016).

Due to their high fiber content, plantains improve your digestive health and help in weight management since they fill you up faster and take longer to digest. Due to their antioxidants content, they protect your body against cell damage from free radicals. Their vitamin C could also help reduce the risks of developing certain forms of cancer. The high amount of potassium contained in plantains also help you maintain a healthy heart while lowering blood pressure and cholesterol.

Plantains are healthy complex carbs with lots of vitamins and minerals, but are normally cooked in lots of grease, or served with heavy cream. If you are choosing to eat healthy, you can opt to just grill or bake them but at the same time let their flavor shine.

Servings: 6

Calories: 182

Carbs: 28 grams

Protein: 1 gram

Fat: 10 grams

Ingredients:

→ 3 cups chopped, ripe plantains

→ ¼ cup coconut oil

→ 1 tbsp cinnamon

→ Sea salt

Directions:

1. Slice a peeled plantain into small pieces.

2. Heat the coconut oil in a pan on low-medium heat. Once hot, add the sliced plantains. Cover and let it cook for about 6 to 7 minutes.

3. Flip the plantains over, cover and cook for another 3 minutes.

4. Sprinkle with cinnamon and sea salt and mix with a spatula, making sure pieces are evenly coated. Let it cool before serving.

High Carb

The Recovery Sandwich

Prep time: 5 minutes

Cook time: 5 minutes

This sandwich will fill you up and help you recover after a long run or some other intense activity. It provides you with the essential macronutrients you need to refuel: carbohydrates to restore your glycogen levels, protein to repair your muscles and fats for many of your essential body and brain functions. This sandwich also has electrolytes and will restore the magnesium, sodium, potassium and chloride levels in your body.

Servings: 1

Calories: 365

Carbs: 59.7 grams

Protein: 19.2 grams

Fat: 9.2 grams

Ingredients:

→ 2 tsp capers

→ ½ ball of mozzarella or 1 cup of cottage cheese

→ 2 tbsp olives

→ ¼ cup sun-dried tomatoes in oil

→ Salt and pepper

→ ¼ cup fresh basil or 1 tsp dried basil

→ 4 slices of whole wheat bread

Directions:

1.   Chop the capers, cheese, olives, and tomatoes into bite size pieces and place in a bowl. Mix together along with the salt, pepper and basil.

2. Mash the ingredients a little bit to release the flavors.

3. Toast the bread.

4. Cover the bottom bread slice with the spread. Place the second slice on top and cover that with the spread. Place the third slice on top and cover that with the spread and place the last slice on top. Flatten the sandwich a bit to compress it and make it easier to heat up in the pan.

5. Preheat your frying pan. Once hot enough, place the sandwich in it and cook for 3 to 4 minutes, flattening the sandwich occasionally. If you have a lid for your frying pan, place the lid on top to let the hot air circulate and cook the sandwich from all sides.

6. Flip over and repeat for the other side.

Shrimp and Lemon Pasta

Prep time: 5 minutes

Cook time: 15 minutes

Are you usually famished after your high-intensity workout? Try this shrimp and lemon pasta to refill our energy tank and help repair your muscles. The protein used for this dish is shrimp, which is low in calories compared to chicken. Aside from providing protein, shrimp offers 100 percent of your daily dose of selenium. This mineral boosts your immunity and thyroid function, while fighting cell damage from free radicals. It also has more than 75 percent of your needed vitamin B12, more than half your phosphorus, and more than 30 percent of your iodine, copper and choline. Shrimp also contains antioxidants, unusual for proteins from animals, that help reduce inflammation. Shrimp however is high in cholesterol so if you already have high levels, it's best to talk to your doctor about adding it to your diet.

Servings: 4

Calories: 430

Carbs: 56 grams

Protein: 35 grams

Fat: 10 grams

Ingredients:

→ 1 tbsp olive oil

→ 1 ½ pounds raw shrimp, peeled and deveined

→ 4 ½ cups of low sodium chicken broth

→ 10 ounces wheat linguine

→ 1 tbsp of any dried herbs (basil, oregano, etc.)

→ 1 ½ cups halved cherry tomatoes

→ 4 tbsp lemon zest

→ ½ cup Kalamata olives

→ 4 cups raw spinach

→ Sea salt & pepper

Directions:

1. Pour the olive oil in a pan and heat on high. Once hot, add the shrimp and cook until it is pink (about 5-7 minutes). Remove from heat and set aside.

2. Lower the heat on the pan to medium and add the chicken broth, linguine, dried herbs, cherry tomatoes, lemon zest and olives. Let it simmer, stirring continuously so the pasta doesn't stick to the pot. Once the pasta is cooked to desired tenderness, lower the heat.

3. Add the spinach and the shrimp. Turn off heat once the spinach leaves wilt.

4. Season with salt and pepper. You may also squeeze some lemon juice onto the pasta.

Banana Muffins

Prep time: 30 minutes

Cook time: 30 minutes

These muffins are lower carb and have fewer calories due to the use of oatmeal flour to replace the usual wheat flour. We are also going to use coconut sugar instead of white sugar. Coconut sugar has a lower GI than white sugar, so it will not cause your blood sugar to spike.

While we make it a practice to use less sugar, what would be a good added sugar that is the lesser of all evils? Coconut sugar may be the answer. This has recently started becoming more popular being touted as a "healthier" alternative to white sugar or high-fructose corn syrup. Coconut sugar is made from coconut tree sap. It is mixed with water to make a syrup, then dried to crystallize. Compared to white sugar and high-fructose corn syrup, this sugar has more calcium, zinc, and iron. It also has small amounts of antioxidants and phytonutrients. Despite these advantages, coconut sugar is still high in simple carbohydrates and calories. If your goal is to lose weight and keep your blood sugar levels stable, it would be best to use it sparingly.

Servings: 8

Calories: 377

Carbs: 44 grams

Protein: 5 grams

Fat: 21 grams

Ingredients:

→ 4 mashed bananas

→ 1 sliced banana

→ 2 cups of oatmeal

→ 1 egg
→ 2 egg whites
→ ⅓ cup coconut oil
→ ⅓ cup coconut sugar
→ 1 tbsp cinnamon
→ 1 ¼ cup coconut milk
→ ½ cup coconut sugar
→ 1 tsp vanilla extract
→ Spray coconut oil

Directions:

1. Preheat your oven to 350°F.

2. Pour oatmeal into a food processor and pulverize it until it is as fine as flour.

3. In a bowl, combine the mashed bananas, eggs, coconut oil, coconut sugar and cinnamon. Mix well.

4. Add the oatmeal flour to the banana mixture and mix well.

5. Spray pan with coconut oil and add coconut milk, coconut sugar and vanilla extract. Cook on high heat for 15 to 20 minutes, then let it cool. The mixture will thicken during this process.

6. Pour the coconut milk mixture into muffin tins, then add the banana slices then the batter.

7. Place the muffins in the oven and cook for 30 minutes. Let the muffins cool slightly before removing them from the tin.

APPENDIX : RECIPES INDEX

B

Bacon & Eggs 50
Baked Eggs With Tex-Mex Beef
Casserole 52
Banana Egg Pancakes 62
Banana Muffins 104
Banana Waffles 56

C

Carrot Cake Protein Oatmeal 66
Carrot, Ginger and Lentil Soup 78
Char Siu Beef With Broccolini 84
Cheesy Chicken and Rice 67
Chickpea Flour Pancakes 60

D

Dutch Apple Pancake 63

E

Easy Granola 90

F

Frittata With Spinach 54

H

Harira 75
Heavy Breakfast With Fried Eggs
and Yogurt 58

I

Indian Chicken Skillet 71

I

Ironman Oatmeal 65

L

Lentil and Brown Rice Salad 82

P

Parmesan Cheese Chips 93
Pea and Ham Soup With Salami
Pesto Puff Pastry 80
Peanut Butter Coconut Cookies 96
Plantains With Cinnamon 98

S

Sake Chicken With Buckwheat
Noodles 86
Salt and Vinegar Zucchini Chips 88
Santa Fe Chicken 69
Sesame Ginger Beef With Noodles
73
Shrimp and Lemon Pasta 102
Soft Pretzels 94
Strawberry Cream Cheese Cups 92

T

The Recovery Sandwich 100

CPSIA information can be obtained
at www.ICGtesting.com
Printed in the USA
LVHW051910090223
739132LV00031B/608